T0226794

Palliative Care in Surgical Oncology

Editor

BRIDGET N. FAHY

SURGICAL ONCOLOGY CLINICS OF NORTH AMERICA

www.surgonc.theclinics.com

Consulting Editor
TIMOTHY M. PAWLIK

July 2021 • Volume 30 • Number 3

ELSEVIER

1600 John F. Kennedy Boulevard • Suite 1800 • Philadelphia, Pennsylvania, 19103-2899

http://www.theclinics.com

SURGICAL ONCOLOGY CLINICS OF NORTH AMERICA Volume 30, Number 3
July 2021 ISSN 1055-3207, ISBN-13: 978-0-323-79061-1

Editor: John Vassallo (j.vassallo@elsevier.com)
Developmental Editor: Diana Ang

Surgical Oncology Clinics of North America (ISSN 1055-3207) is published quarterly by Elsevier Inc., 360 Park Avenue South, New York, NY 10010-1710. Months of publication are January, April, July, and October. Business and Editorial Offices: 1600 John F. Kennedy Blvd., Ste. 1800, Philadelphia, PA 19103-2899. Customer Service Office: 3251 Riverport Lane, Maryland Heights, MO 63043. Periodicals postage paid at New York, NY and additional mailing offices. Subscription prices are $315.00 per year (US individuals), $750.00 (US institutions) $100.00 (US student/resident), $352.00 (Canadian individuals), $784.00 (Canadian institutions), $100.00 (Canadian student/resident), $456.00 (foreign individuals), $784.00 (foreign institutions), and $205.00 (foreign student/resident). Foreign air speed delivery is included in all *Clinics* subscription prices. All prices are subject to change without notice. **POSTMASTER**: Send address changes to *Surgical Oncology Clinics of North America*, Elsevier Health Science Division, Subscription Customer Service, 3251 Riverport Lane, Maryland Heights, MO 63043. **Customer Service: 1-800-654-2452 (US and Canada). 314-447-8871 (outside US and Canada). Fax: 314-447-8029. E-mail: journalscustomerservice-usa@elsevier.com (for print support); journalsonline support-usa@elsevier.com (for online support).**

Reprints. For copies of 100 or more, of articles in this publication, please contact the Commercial Reprints Department, Elsevier Inc., 360 Park Avenue South, New York, New York 10010-1710. Tel. 212-633-3874; Fax: 212-633-3820; E-mail: reprints@elsevier.com.

Surgical Oncology Clinics of North America is covered in *MEDLINE/PubMed (Index Medicus)* and *EMBASE/ Excerpta Medica, Current Contents/Clinical Medicine, and ISI/BIOMED.*

Contributors

CONSULTING EDITOR

TIMOTHY M. PAWLIK, MD, MPH, MTS, PhD, FACS, FRACS (Hon.)
Professor and Chair, Department of Surgery, The Urban Meyer III and Shelley Meyer Chair for Cancer Research, Professor of Surgery, Oncology, Health Services Management and Policy, Surgeon in Chief, The Ohio State University Wexner Medical Center, Columbus, Ohio, USA

EDITOR

BRIDGET N. FAHY, MD
Department of Surgery, Division of Surgical Oncology, University of New Mexico, Division of Palliative Medicine, University of New Mexico, Albuquerque, New Mexico, USA

AUTHORS

JOSH BLEICHER, MD MS
Division of General Surgery, Huntsman Cancer Institute, University of Utah, Salt Lake City, Utah, USA

BENOIT BLONDEAU, MD, MBA, FACS
Department of Surgery, Division of Trauma Surgery, Division of Palliative Medicine, University of New Mexico, Albuquerque, New Mexico, USA

ANISH A. BUTALA, MD
Department of Radiation Oncology, Hospital of the University of Pennsylvania, Perelman Center for Advanced Medicine, Philadelphia, Pennsylvania, USA

BRIDGET N. FAHY, MD
Department of Surgery, Division of Surgical Oncology, University of New Mexico, Division of Palliative Medicine, University of New Mexico, Albuquerque, New Mexico, USA

ESMÉFINLAY, MD
Associate Professor, Department of Internal Medicine, Division of Palliative Medicine, University of New Mexico School of Medicine, The University of New Mexico Health Sciences Center, Albuquerque, New Mexico, USA

NADIA V. GUARDADO, MD
Department of Surgery, University of New Mexico School of Medicine, Albuquerque, New Mexico, USA

BREANA L. HILL, MD
Department of Obstetrics and Gynecology, University of Colorado School of Medicine, Aurora, Colorado, USA

ALEXANDRA C. ISTL, MD, MPH
Clinical Fellow, Division of Surgical Oncology, Johns Hopkins Hospital, Baltimore, Maryland, USA

FABIAN M. JOHNSTON, MD, MHS
Associate Professor, Division of Surgical Oncology, Johns Hopkins Hospital, Baltimore, Maryland, USA

JOSHUA A. JONES, MD, MA, FAAHPM
Assistant Professor, Department of Radiation Oncology, Hospital of the University of Pennsylvania, Perelman Center for Advanced Medicine, Philadelphia, Pennsylvania, USA

LAURA A. LAMBERT, MD
Division of General Surgery, Huntsman Cancer Institute, University of Utah, Salt Lake City, Utah, USA

CAROLYN LEFKOWITS, MD
Department of Obstetrics and Gynecology, Division of Gynecologic Oncology, University of Colorado School of Medicine, Aurora, Colorado, USA

ELIZABETH J. LILLEY, MD, MPH
Center for Surgery and Public Health at Brigham and Women's Hospital, Department of Psychosocial Oncology and Palliative Care, Dana-Farber Cancer Institute, Division of Palliative Care and Geriatric Medicine, Department of Medicine, Massachusetts General Hospital, Boston, Massachusetts, USA

KAYSEY LLORENTE, MD
Department of Surgery, University of New Mexico School of Medicine, Albuquerque, New Mexico, USA

SHWETHA H. MANJUNATH, MD
Department of Radiation Oncology, Hospital of the University of Pennsylvania, Perelman Center for Advanced Medicine, Philadelphia, Pennsylvania, USA

SUSAN McCAMMON, MFA, MD, FACS
John W. Poynor Professor in Otolaryngology, Professor, Department of Otolaryngology–Head and Neck Surgery, Department of Internal Medicine, Division of Gerontology, Geriatrics, and Palliative Care, Assistant Director, Community-Based Palliative Care, UAB Center for Palliative and Supportive Care, The University of Alabama at Birmingham, Birmingham, Alabama, USA

SHAILA J. MERCHANT, MSc, MHSc, MD, FRCSC
Associate Professor, Division of General Surgery and Surgical Oncology, Queen's University, Kingston, Ontario, Canada

THOMAS J. MINER, MD, FACS
Department of Surgery, Rhode Island Hospital, Warren Alpert Medical School of Brown University, Providence, Rhode Island, USA

ALYSSA K. OVAITT, MD
Department of Otolaryngology–Head and Neck Surgery, The University of Alabama at Birmingham, Birmingham, Alabama, USA

CASSANDRA S. PARKER, MD
Department of Surgery, Rhode Island Hospital, Warren Alpert Medical School of Brown University, Providence, Rhode Island, USA

RAMSES SAAVEDRA, MD
Department of Surgery, University of New Mexico School of Medicine, Albuquerque, New Mexico, USA

LORI SPOOZAK, MD, MHS, FACOG, FACS
Associate Professor of Obstetrics and Gynecology, Divisions of Gynecologic Oncology and Palliative Medicine, University of Kansas Medical Center, Kansas City, Kansas, USA

GRAEME R. WILLIAMS, MD, MBA
Department of Radiation Oncology, Hospital of the University of Pennsylvania, Perelman Center for Advanced Medicine, Leonard Davis Institute of Healthcare Economics, University of Pennsylvania, Philadelphia, Pennsylvania, USA

ELIZABETH WULFF-BURCHFIELD, MD
Assistant Professor of Internal Medicine, Divisions of Medical Oncology and Palliative Medicine, University of Kansas Medical Center, Kansas City, Kansas, USA; University of Kansas Medical Center, Westwood, Kansas, USA

CAITLIN T. YEO, BSc, MD
Surgical Oncology Fellow, Division of Surgical Oncology, University of Calgary, Calgary, Alberta, Canada

Contents

> Multiple cancer societies and professional medical organizations recommend integration of palliative care into routine oncology care. A growing body of literature supports the benefits of palliative care in patients with cancer. Palliative care improves pain and other symptoms, enhances quality of life, and reduces depression. The best method and timing for integration of palliative care is unclear. Multiple barriers exist that prevent optimal palliative care integration; these barriers will require additional education and research to overcome.

> Surgical palliation in oncology can be defined as "procedures employed with non-curative intent with the primary goal of improving symptoms caused by an advanced malignancy," and is an important aspect of the end-of-life care of patients with incurable malignancies. Palliative interventions may provide great benefit, but they also carry high risk for morbidity and mortality, which may be minimized with careful patient selection. This can be done by consideration of the patient and his or her indication for the given intervention via open communication, as well as prediction of benefits and risks to define the therapeutic index of the operation or procedure.

> Malignant bowel obstruction is a challenging clinical problem encountered in patients with advanced abdominal and pelvic malignancies. Although medical therapies form the foundation of management, some patients may be suitable candidates for surgical and procedural interventions. The literature is composed primarily of retrospective single-institution experiences and the results of prospective trials are pending. Given the high symptom burden and limited life expectancy of these patients, management may be best informed by multidisciplinary teams with relevant expertise.

In addition to severe, life-limiting complications such as malignant bowel obstruction, fistulae, and malignant ascites, peritoneal carcinomatosis frequently causes life-impacting symptoms such as pain, nausea, anorexia, cachexia, and fatigue. A variety of medical, interventional, and surgical therapies are now available for management of both complications and symptoms. Although surgery in this population is often associated with a relatively high risk of morbidity and mortality, operative intervention can offer effective palliative treatment in appropriately selected patients. Early involvement of palliative care specialists as part of a multidisciplinary team is essential to providing optimal, holistic care of patients with peritoneal carcinomatosis.

There is no reason to be pollyannaish when approaching patients with malignant biliary obstruction (MBO). Although technology has allowed refining diagnosis and resectability of cancers causing biliary obstruction, outcomes have not improved significantly. The previous preponderant place of surgical procedures now is replaced by endoluminal and percutaneous techniques for the management of symptoms of MBO. Because quantity of life often is the primary and sole outcome for evaluation of various interventions, the main focus of patient quality of life may be erroneously deemphasized. Lagging behind scientific advances are the availability of palliative care services and studies of patient-related outcomes.

Cancer is a progressive disease that can lead to malnutrition and cachexia. Artificial nutrition is a medical therapy used to combat malnutrition in these patients. In this article, the authors discuss factors affecting the decision to use artificial nutrition, including the patient's mental and physical health, technical factors of the procedures used to deliver artificial nutrition, and the oncologic factors affecting treatment. Through this review, the authors provide guidelines on who is and is not likely to benefit from therapy, available routes of administration, and necessary factors to consider for appropriate decision-making for palliative patients and those with advanced cancers."

Effective management of pain in patients with cancer impacts quality of life and willingness to receive disease-directed treatment. This review focuses on preoperative, intraoperative, and postoperative strategies for management of perioperative pain in the patient with cancer. Managing perioperative pain in special populations, including patients with preoperative opioid use, those with a history of substance abuse, and patients near the end of life are also addressed.

The importance of integrated palliative care in surgical oncology has been established by high-level evidence demonstrating improved patient-centered outcomes. There has been substantial improvement in efforts to incorporate palliative medicine training into medical and surgical education over the last decade. However, although trainees may feel confident in managing patients at the end of life, they may not have the insight or proficiency to provide optimal palliative care. Surgeons and palliative care physicians should collaborate on methods to optimize palliative care education for both trainees and practicing surgeons. A growing number of palliative care resources are available to this end.

SURGICAL ONCOLOGY
CLINICS OF NORTH AMERICA

FORTHCOMING ISSUES

October 2021
Management of Pancreatic Cancer
Susan Tsai and Douglas B. Evans, *Editors*

January 2022
Disparities and Determinants of Health in Surgical Oncology
Oluwadamilola "Lola" Fayanju, *Editor*

April 2022
Colorectal Cancer
Traci L. Hedrick, *Editor*

RECENT ISSUES

April 2021
Pediatric Cancer
Roshni Dasgupta, *Editor*

January 2021
Management of Metastatic Liver Tumors
Michael D'Angelica, *Editor*

October 2020
Emerging Therapies in Thoracic Malignancies
Usman Ahmad and Sudish C. Murthy, *Editors*

SERIES OF RELATED INTEREST

Surgical Clinics of North America
http://www.surgical.theclinics.com
Thoracic Surgery Clinics
http://www.thoracic.theclinics.com
Advances in Surgery
http://www.advancessurgery.com

THE CLINICS ARE AVAILABLE ONLINE!
Access your subscription at:
www.theclinics.com

Foreword

Palliative Care in Surgical Oncology

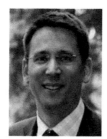

Timothy M. Pawlik, MD, MPH, MTS, PhD, FACS, FRACS (Hon.)
Consulting Editor

This issue of the *Surgical Oncology Clinics of North America* focuses on Palliative Care in Surgical Oncology. The World Health Organization defines palliative care as "an approach that improves the quality of life of patients and their families facing the problems associated with life-threatening illness, through the prevention and relief of suffering by means of early identification and impeccable assessment and treatment of pain and other problems, physical, psychosocial, and spiritual."[1] Palliative care improves the quality of life of patients and that of their families who are facing challenges associated with life-threatening illness, whether physical, psychological, social, or spiritual. Palliative care involves a range of services delivered by a wide scope of professionals, including physicians, nurses, pharmacists, physiotherapists, and volunteers, that all have important roles to play in supporting the patient and their family. In a discipline such as oncology, palliative care has particular relevance. Many patients with cancer are in need relief of symptoms, pain, and the existential stress of a cancer diagnosis that may be life-limiting. As such, the integration of palliative care needs to be "best practice" in oncology—not only at the end of life but also throughout the entire patient care journey. Concurrent with the increased recognition of the importance of palliative care in oncologic care, there has been a growing body of academic scholarship focused on the impact of palliative care in the care of patients with cancer. In light of this, I am grateful to have Dr Bridget N. Fahy, MD as the guest editor of this important issue of *Surgical Oncology Clinics of North America*. Dr Fahy is professor and chief of the Division of Surgical Oncology in the Department of Surgery at the University of New Mexico (UNM) School of Medicine. She is the medical coordinator of the UNM Comprehensive Cancer Center's surgical services and Professor of Internal Medicine in the Division of Palliative Medicine. Dr Fahy completed her general surgery training at University of California, Davis and her surgical oncology training at Memorial Sloan Kettering Cancer Center. Dr Fahy is board certified in Hospice and Palliative Medicine

Surg Oncol Clin N Am 30 (2021) xiii–xiv
https://doi.org/10.1016/j.soc.2021.03.003
1055-3207/21/© 2021 Published by Elsevier Inc.

and currently serves as the UNM Medical Director of Surgical Palliative Care. As such, Dr Fahy is extremely well qualified to be the guest editor of this issue of *Surgical Oncology Clinics of North America*.

The issue covers a number of important topics, including selecting patients for palliative procedures, as well as approaches to malignant bowel obstruction, peritoneal carcinomatosis, and strategies for optimizing perioperative pain management for the patient with cancer. In addition, other important topics, such as how to navigate difficult discussions, breaking bad news, and a detailed overview of the ethical considerations in caring for patients with advanced malignancy, are provided. The wide range of topics, as well as the depth covered in each article, presents the readers with an unparalleled opportunity to learn about the role of palliative care in surgical oncology.

I am very grateful to Dr Fahy for her efforts in identifying such a notable group of co-authors who are leaders in the field of palliative care to contribute to this issue of *Surgical Oncology Clinics of North America*. Collectively, the authors have done a superb job emphasizing the various aspects of caring for patients with cancer and the importance of integrating palliative care into our clinical practice. In a discipline that frequently confronts both patients and providers with challenging clinical, ethical, and existential matters, this issue of *Surgical Oncology Clinics of North America* will serve faculty and trainees well. My hope is that readers of *Surgical Oncology Clinics of North America* will find value in this issue and that these concepts are readily applicable to their clinical practice. Once again, I would like to thank Dr Fahy and all the contributing authors for this exceptional issue of the *Surgical Oncology Clinics of North America*.

Timothy M. Pawlik, MD, MPH, MTS, PhD, FACS, FRACS (Hon.)
Department of Surgery
The Urban Meyer III and Shelley Meyer Chair for Cancer Research
Departments of Surgery, Oncology, and Health Services Management and Policy
The Ohio State University Wexner Medical Center
395 West 12th Avenue, Suite 670
Columbus, OH 43210, USA

E-mail address:
tim.pawlik@osumc.edu

REFERENCE

1. WHO. Definition of palliative care, 2008. World Health Organization. Available at: http://www.who.int/cancer/palliative/definition/en/. Accessed March 22, 2021.

Preface

Understanding the Surgeons' Role in Palliation of the Oncology Patient

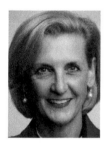

Bridget N. Fahy, MD
Editor

Much has changed since the last issue of *Surgical Oncology Clinics of North America* was devoted to the topic of palliative surgical oncology in 2004. That issue, guest edited by Dr Lawrence Wagman with consulting editor Dr Nicholas Petrelli, focused on many of the key issues of surgical palliative care in oncology, including unique aspects related to palliation of various malignancies and surgical management of malignant bowel obstruction. As Dr Petrelli astutely noted in his foreword to the issue, "I would have to say that this issue is probably the most important for surgical oncology fellows to read. These physicians, after completing their fellowship training, will be faced with issues related to palliative surgical oncology care throughout their careers. It is also important for trainees in the disciplines of medical and radiation oncology to be familiar with these concepts to be able to consult with a surgeon at the appropriate time, not when there is no chance for improving quality of life." Dr Petrelli's comments are as true today as they were in 2004.

What has changed in the intervening 16 years is a growing appreciation of the need for palliation from the time of cancer diagnosis through end of life. This appreciation is manifest by the creation of Hospice and Palliative Medicine as a medical subspecialty in 2006. The American Board of Surgery was among the 10 cosponsoring boards of certification in this new subspecialty. In addition, a palliative care standard was incorporated in 2012 as part of the standards of quality, comprehensive cancer care by the Commission on Cancer.

Coupled with enhanced understanding of the role of palliative medicine in conjunction with cancer-directed therapies is a growing body of literature illustrating the benefits of early palliative care in oncology. As central providers of cancer care, surgeons must be able to incorporate this knowledge into their daily surgical practice. In

Surg Oncol Clin N Am 30 (2021) xv–xvi
https://doi.org/10.1016/j.soc.2021.03.004
1055-3207/21/© 2021 Published by Elsevier Inc.

surgonc.theclinics.com

addition, there is a critical need for research that addresses the unique needs of surgical oncology patients to ensure that they receive not just state-of-the-art cancer care but also the kind of patient-centered, whole-person care that is the foundation of palliative care.

The current issue draws on the expertise of an all-star group of surgeons, medical oncologists, and radiation oncologists who address the spectrum of palliative care issues that face oncology providers on a routine basis. In addition to their unique oncology expertise, the authors also represent national thought-leaders in the field of palliative medicine. Many of the articles tackle common challenges, such as management of malignant bowel obstruction, peritoneal carcinomatosis and malignant ascites, malignant biliary obstruction, and guidelines for selecting patients for palliative procedures in oncology. In addition, the authors provide practical approaches to the use of artificial nutrition in patients with advanced malignancy, palliative chemotherapy and radiotherapy, ethical considerations in patients with advanced malignancy, and navigating difficult conversations in oncology. This special issue also includes an article dedicated to the role of palliative medicine training in surgical oncology, reflecting the critical, and unfortunately often unmet, need for education specifically related to palliative medicine.

It has been my pleasure and privilege to serve as the guest editor for this special issue on Palliative Care in Surgical Oncology. I am indebted to my fellow authors for sharing their expertise, which, I am certain, will be of significant value to our readers and their patients.

Bridget N. Fahy, MD
Department of Surgery
University of New Mexico
1 University of New Mexico, MSC 07-4025
Albuquerque, NM 87131, USA

E-mail address:
bfahy@salud.unm.edu

Current Guidelines for Integration of Palliative Care in Oncology

Bridget N. Fahy, MD[a,b]

KEYWORDS

- Palliative care • Oncology • Symptom management • Quality of life

KEY POINTS

- Palliative care is as an essential component of cancer care.
- All patients should be screened for palliative care needs at the time of diagnosis and at regular intervals throughout the course of routine cancer care, as well at end of life.
- Palliative care has been shown to reduce the burden of symptoms, enhance quality of life, and improve mood.
- Receipt of palliative care may impact health care resource use in patients with cancer, particularly at end of life.
- Significant barriers exist that prevent integration of palliative care into routine cancer care with unique barriers for surgical oncology patients.

INTRODUCTION

Palliative cancer and oncology are inextricably linked. The term palliative care was introduced in 1974 by Balfour Mount, a surgical oncologist, at the Royal Victoria Hospital of McGill University in Montreal, Canada. The close ties between palliative care and cancer reflect a recognition that palliative care is needed in patients with life-limiting illnesses, such as cancer, both during and following cancer-directed therapies. According to the World Health Organization, patients with cancer account for approximately one-third of all patients in need of palliative care, second only to those with cardiovascular disease.[1]

The current guidelines for integrating palliative care with cancer care reflect an evolution in the understanding of what palliative care is, and is not. Most notably, the erroneous equation between palliative care and end-of-life care continues to be a stubborn misperception. Palliative medicine is a multidisciplinary and

^a Department of Surgery, Division of Surgical Oncology, University of New Mexico, 1 University of New Mexico, MSC 07-4025, Albuquerque, NM 87131, USA; ^b Division of Palliative Medicine, University of New Mexico, Albuquerque, NM, USA
E-mail address: bfahy@salud.unm.edu

Surg Oncol Clin N Am 30 (2021) 431–447
https://doi.org/10.1016/j.soc.2021.02.002
1055-3207/21/© 2021 Elsevier Inc. All rights reserved.

interdisciplinary medical specialty that addresses several distinct domains: physical, psychological, social, spiritual/religious/existential, cultural, as well as end-of-life care.[2] Although it incorporates these same domains, hospice care is appropriate for patients with a life expectancy of 6 months or less if a disease takes its expected course. With rare exceptions, hospice care is not appropriate for patients whose goal is life prolongation, particularly through receipt of cancer-directed therapies that are not strictly palliative. Despite the early introduction of palliative care into cancer care advocated by Dr Mount in the 1970s, the progress toward realization of his vision has been slow. Only recently have national oncology organizations and professional societies made a more concerted effort to encourage providers to routinely integrate palliative care into standard cancer care. In addition to the perceptual progress made, advances in palliative care integration into cancer care are the result of a growing body of research focused on the impact of palliative care for patients with cancer at all stages of disease, including those receiving curative-intent treatments.

The following discussion reviews the current guidelines for integrating palliative care into standard oncology care as published by several national oncology organizations and professional societies, and summarizes some of the key evidence on which the current guidelines are based. Barriers to integration of palliative care into usual cancer care are noted, as well efforts needed to address these barriers. In addition, recommendations for integrating palliative care into oncology are made with a specific note of needs for surgical oncology patients.

PROFESSIONAL ORGANIZATIONS ADDRESS NEED FOR PALLIATIVE CARE IN PATIENTS WITH CANCER
American Society of Clinical Oncology

The American Society of Clinical Oncology (ASCO) first broached the topic of palliative care for oncology patients by focusing on patients at end of life. In their article entitled "Cancer Care During the Last Phase of Life," the investigators advocated for hospice as an excellent model for managing end-of-life care and thought this required access to state-of-the-art palliative care provided by skilled clinicians, with palliative care experts, as needed.[3] The synonymous usage of hospice and palliative care continued by ASCO (and most other professional medical organizations) for almost a decade before a distinction between end-of-life care and palliative care was significantly appreciated. The false equivalence of these 2 related but distinct forms of medical care was responsible, in part, for delayed integration of palliative care with oncology care. It was not until 2009 that ASCO formally introduced the concept of integrating palliative care throughout the course of cancer care.[4] In 2012, ASCO published a provisional clinical opinion on the integration of palliative care in oncology based on a review of the available clinical trials that, for the first time, provided strong evidence to support concurrent palliative care with standard oncology care.[5] A clinical practice guideline update was published in 2016 based on updated systematic reviews, randomized clinical trials, and metaanalyses.[6] The investigators sought to answer the question of whether palliative care concurrent with oncology care should be standard practice. Their summary recommendation was, "Patients with advanced cancer, whether in-patient or outpatient, should receive dedicated palliative care services, early in the disease course, concurrent with active treatment. Referring patients to interdisciplinary palliative care teams is optimal, and services may complement existing programs."[6]

Society of Surgical Oncology

The Society of Surgical Oncology (SSO), as part of the American Federation of Clinical Oncologic Societies, first endorsed palliative and supportive care as a component of quality cancer care in 1998.[7] As part of this consensus statement, the sponsoring societies agreed that "Supportive care services and effective symptom management are essential to promoting the quality of life for people diagnosed with cancer. Patients must have access to these services and therapies as part of their comprehensive cancer care."[7] Since this initial statement, the SSO has not provided any further statements on the role of palliative care in oncology. In a recent editorial by Brian Badgwell,[8] he surmises that the lack of further guidance from the SSO reflects an understanding that SSO guidance fits under the ASCO statement. In the absence of any explicit statements on the integration of palliative care for surgical oncology patients, the SSO's intent on this topic can only be inferred.

Institute of Medicine

The Institute of Medicine (IOM) has published several statements about the role of palliative care as a component of comprehensive cancer care, beginning in 1997. Similar to ASCO, the early focus of these statements was on end-of-life care.[9] Two years later, the IOM published another report *Ensuring Quality Cancer Care*, in which they recommended that guidelines based on the best available evidence be developed for (cancer) prevention, diagnosis, treatment, and palliative care.[10] The significance of including palliative care along with other standard aspects of cancer care cannot be overemphasized, because this guideline was among the first to emphasize the need to integrate palliative care into standard cancer care. In 2001, the IOM published *Improving Palliative Care for Cancer*, in which the investigators made 10 recommendations on various aspects of palliative care in oncology, which included development of a core set of cancer quality measures as they pertain to palliative care, requirements for recognition of a comprehensive cancer center, ensuring access to information about palliative care through various patient-oriented organizations, and the need for research in palliative care.[11] Since this 2001 publication, the National Academies of Science, Engineering, and Medicine has published numerous other proceedings and consensus reports about the importance of, and guidelines for, integrating palliative care into cancer care for both children and adults.[12]

American College of Surgeons, Commission on Cancer

The Commission on Cancer (CoC) was established by the American College of Surgeons (ACS) in 1922 to establish standards to ensure quality, comprehensive cancer care. The palliative care Standard 2.4 was introduced in 2012, with CoC-accredited centers required to meet this standard by 2015.[13] This standard was part of new patient-centered functions and quality measurement and outcomes. Standard 2.4 required CoC-accredited centers to have palliative care services available to patients either on site or by referral. The availability of palliative care services was identified as an essential component of cancer care, beginning at the diagnosis and being continuously available throughout treatment, surveillance, and, when applicable, during bereavement. The palliative care standard was updated in 2016 to include emphasis that palliative care was not simply hospice care, again reinforcing the role of introducing palliative care services from the time of diagnosis and not only at end of life.[14] The CoC 2020 standards continue to include a palliative care standard (now Standard 4.5); it includes a requirement that programs evaluate palliative care use, criteria for referral, and areas for improvement.[15]

National Comprehensive Cancer Network

The National Comprehensive Cancer Network (NCCN) first published guidelines on the integration of palliative care into cancer care in 2003.[16] Since then, the guidelines have been updated and expanded on an annual basis. The most current NCCN palliative care guidelines include several standards of palliative care,[17] including:

- Institutions should develop processes for integrating palliative care into cancer care, both as part of usual oncology care and for patients with specialty palliative care needs.
- All patients with cancer should be screened for palliative care needs after initial visit, at appropriate intervals, and as clinically indicated.
- Patients/family/caregivers should be informed that palliative care is an integral part of their comprehensive cancer care.

In addition, the current guidelines contain a robust set of recommendations on topics ranging from indications for palliative care specialist consultation to management of several common symptoms (eg, pain, dyspnea, constipation) to advance care planning to palliative sedation. A detailed review of all palliative care–related guidelines contained within the most recent version of the NCCN guidelines is beyond the scope of this article. As with all NCCN guidelines, they are a statement of evidence and consensus of the investigators regarding their views of currently accepted approaches to treatment. Notably absent from the current guidelines is representation of a surgical oncologist on the NCCN palliative care panel or any specific guidance regarding selection of patients for palliative surgical intervention.

WHAT IS THE EVIDENCE FOR INTEGRATING PALLIATIVE CARE INTO CANCER CARE?

As outlined earlier, the earliest discussions about the role of palliative care in patients with cancer focused on patients at end of life, specifically when cancer treatment was no longer provided. One of the earliest studies to examine the impact of palliative care in patients with terminal cancer was published by Higginson and McCarthy[18] in 1989. The investigators examined changes in symptoms of 86 patients referred to a terminal care support team and found significant improvements in pain after 1 week of care, with further improvement into the week of death. Several studies have subsequently been published that examined the impact of palliative care on patients with cancer who received palliative care services in various settings (inpatient, home based). Most of these early studies prospectively studied patients who received various palliative care interventions. Most, but not all, studies found an improvement in pain and nonpain symptoms, overall quality of life, and mood in patients following receipt of the palliative care intervention.

Coincident with the increased focus on earlier introduction of palliative care in the late 2000s came the introduction of clinical trials designed to assess the impact of providing palliative care concurrent with cancer care. Integrated or early palliative care are the terms most often used to describe the simultaneous provision of palliative care with cancer-directed therapies. The seminal randomized clinical trial evaluating the impact of integrated palliative care was published by Temel and colleagues[19] in 2010. The investigators randomized patients with newly diagnosed metastatic non–small-cell lung cancer (NSCLC) to palliative care integrated with standard oncologic care or standard oncologic care alone. The primary outcome was change in quality of life at 12 weeks. Patients assigned to early palliative care had better quality of life and fewer patients had depressive symptoms. Since this landmark study, numerous studies have been performed to evaluate the impact of palliative care in patients with cancer. These studies have varied by tumor type, stage of disease, and receipt of cancer therapies. Studies have also varied in the specific palliative care interventions provided; some have focused on symptom control, whereas others have addressed quality of life and mood. The setting for provision of palliative care also varies between inpatient, clinic-based, and home-based care. A summary of several key studies on the impact of palliative care on symptoms, quality of life, mood, and other patient-reported outcomes is provided in **Table 1**.

Patient-Reported Outcomes, Symptoms

Pain and nonpain symptoms have reportedly been improved with involvement of palliative care in most of the studies published.[18,20–22,24–28,30,33] Of the studies that did not show an improvement in symptoms in the palliative care intervention group, 1 group hypothesized that there may be little room for improvement when low symptom intensity scores are reported in a given symptom domain.[25] Given the heterogeneity of patients with cancer included in the studies, it is also possible that this variability reflects tumor-related differences in various symptom domains. For example, dyspnea may be a significant symptom for patients with lung cancer but a less prominent symptom for patients with gastrointestinal malignancies. The effect of palliative care intervention for any 1 domain may be obscured by the number of patients with a given tumor represented in the overall patient population studied. The method by which symptoms are assessed also varied by study. In most studies, the Edmonton Symptom Assessment System was the standardized instrument used. However, this was not uniformly used, which may have contributed to the lack of benefit seen in the palliative care intervention arm and at least 2 of the studies.[33,35]

A summary of the effect of palliative care intervention on various individual symptoms is provided in **Table 1**. Pain was the most common symptom assessed in most studies. Patients who received the palliative care intervention had improvement in pain in 7 of the studies reviewed.[18,20–22,24,26,27] The impact of palliative care on several gastrointestinal symptoms, including nausea, anorexia, constipation, and diarrhea, has been reported in multiple studies. Overall, patients receiving palliative care reported an improvement in these symptoms.[20–22,24,26,33] Patients who received palliative care have also shown an improvement in insomnia[20,24,26] and fatigue.[24,26,27] Improvement in dyspnea with palliative care has been less consistent. Two studies found no change in dyspnea scores after the introduction of palliative care,[18,24] whereas other investigators reported improvement[26] or initial improvement followed by worsening in the last days of life.[22] These findings show the complex trajectory and challenges in management of some symptoms experienced by patients with cancer, particularly in the final days of life.

Quality of Life

In addition to symptoms, quality of life is one of the other most commonly assessed domains in the integrated palliative care literature. The most common instrument used is the European Organisation for Research and Treatment of Cancer Quality of Life (EORTC-QLQ) C-30.[38] The generic questionnaire originally developed in 1988 now has 19 specific modules. **Table 1** includes a summary of several key studies that have assessed the impact of palliative care on quality of life in patients with cancer. Of the 14 studies cited, 10 showed a significant improvement in quality of life among patients who received the palliative care intervention. Although improvements in symptom control generally correlated with improvements in overall quality of life, at least 2 studies showed an improvement in quality of life despite a lack of significant impact of palliative care on symptoms.[25,31] Differences in assessment tools used to

Table 1
Impact of palliative care on symptoms, quality of life, and mood

	Care Setting	Study Design	Symptom	QoL	Mood	Other
Higginson & McCarthy,[18] 1989	Hospital and home PCT	N = 86 Retrospective review	↓ Pain; No change in dyspnea	—	—	—
Ellershaw et al,[20] 1995	Hospital PCT	N = 125 Prospective study	↑ Control multiple symptoms	—	—	↑ Diagnostic and prognostic understanding
Peruselli et al,[21] 1997	Home PCT	N = 73 Prospective study	↓ Pain; ↑ Appetite; ↓ Nausea	—	Improved	—
Mercadante et al,[22] 2000	Home PCT	N = 373 Prospective study	↓ Pain; ↓ Nausea/vomiting; ↓ Diarrhea; Initial ↓ dyspnea and constipation	—	—	—
Jordhøy et al,[23] 2001	Cooperation between palliative medicine unit and community service	N = 235 intervention N = 199 controls Cluster randomized trial	—	No difference	—	—
Strömgren et al,[24] 2005	Referrals to PC department	N = 201 Longitudinal assessment	↓ Pain; ↓ Anorexia; ↓ Nausea/vomiting; ↓ Fatigue; ↓ Insomnia; ↓ Constipation; No change in dyspnea	↑	No change in depression; ↓ Anxiety	—
Bakitas et al,[25] 2009	Telephone sessions	N = 161 intervention N = 161 usual care RCT	↓ Symptom intensity (trend)	↑	↓ Depression	—

Study	Setting	N/Design	Symptoms	QoL	Psychological	Other
Follwell et al,[26] 2009	Oncology PC clinic	N = 150 Prospective study	↓ Pain ↓ Fatigue ↓ Nausea ↓ Anorexia ↓ Insomnia ↓ Dyspnea ↓ Constipation	—	↓ Distress ↓ Depression ↓ Anxiety	—
Temel et al,[19] 2010	Outpatient PC	N = 151 Randomized trial	—	↑	↓ Depression	—
Bischoff et al,[27] 2013	Outpatient PC comanagement	N = 266 Observational study	↓ Pain ↓ Fatigue No change in nausea	↑	↓ Depression ↓ Anxiety	↑ Spiritual well-being
Zimmermann et al,[28] 2014	Outpatient PC	N = 228 intervention N = 233 control	Improvement in multiple symptoms at 4 mo.	↑	—	↑ Spiritual well-being
Bakitas et al,[29] 2015	PC telehealth	N = 307 Random assignment of early vs late PC	No difference	No difference	↓ Depression in early PC	—
Ferrell et al,[30] 2015	Outpatient PC	N = 491 Prospective, serial accrual of usual care followed by intervention group	Improvement in symptoms	↑	↓ Psychological distress	↑ Spiritual well-being
Grudzen et al,[31] 2016	Inpatient PC after emergency department referral	N = 69 PC N = 67 usual care RCT	No difference	↑	No difference in depression	—
Maltoni et al,[32] 2016	Outpatient PC	N = 107 systematic PC N = 107 on demand PC Multicenter randomized trial	—	↑	No difference	—

(continued on next page)

Table 1
(continued)

	Care Setting	Study Design	Symptom	QoL	Mood	Other
Groenvold et al,[33] 2017	Outpatient PC	N = 145 PC N = 152 standard care Multicenter randomized trial	No effect on primary need Possible ↓ in nausea/vomiting	—	—	—
Temel et al,[34] 2017	Outpatient PC	N = 175 integrated PC N = 175 usual care Random assignment	—	↑	↓ Depression	—
Johnsen et al,[35] 2020	Outpatient PC	N = 145 integrated PC N = 152 standard care Multicenter randomized trial	No effect on symptoms	No effect	No effect on anxiety or depression	—
Slama et al,[36] 2020	Outpatient PC	N = 60 integrated PC N = 66 standard care RCT	—	No difference	No difference in depression or anxiety	—
Vanbutsele et al,[37] 2020	Outpatient PC	N = 186 Random assignment	—	↑	—	—

Abbreviations: PC, palliative care; PCT, palliative care team; QoL, quality of life; RCT, randomized control trial.

measure quality of life, timing of the palliative care intervention, and definitions of what constitutes significant improvement may contribute to the variable relationship between symptom control and quality of life.

Mood

The impact of palliative care on mood in patients with cancer was reviewed in 13 studies. Unlike assessments of symptoms and quality of life, the instrument used to assess changes in mood with palliative care interventions is less uniform. Depression and anxiety are domains assessed as part of the Edmonton Symptom Assessment System. Emotional function is a domain of the EORTC-QLQ-C30. The other commonly used instrument to assess mood is the Hospital Anxiety and Depression Scale (HADS). Despite these differences in measurements of mood in patients who received palliative care, 9 of the studies reviewed showed an improvement in depression and/or anxiety among patients who received the palliative care intervention. One of the studies that used the HADS instrument found a decreasing trend in emotional distress and anxiety after 2 months of their palliative care intervention; however, the differences did not reach statistical significance and may be attributed to multiple factors, including the short duration of the palliative care intervention.[35]

Spiritual Well-Being

A limited number of studies have assessed the impact of palliative care intervention on spiritual well-being (see **Table 1**). The most widely used instrument is the Functional Assessment of Chronic Illness Therapy-Spiritual Well-Being (FACIT-Sp 12).[39] Bischoff and colleagues,[27] Zimmermann and colleagues,[28] and Ferrell and colleagues[30] found an improvement in spiritual well-being as measured by the FACIT-Sp 12 in patients with cancer who received outpatient palliative care. The details of how the palliative care providers addressed spiritual concerns is unclear. The spiritual needs of patients with cancer as part of a palliative care intervention is a largely untapped area of research.

OTHER OUTCOMES OF INTEGRATED PALLIATIVE CARE IN CANCER

The beneficial impact of palliative care integration with usual cancer care on pain and nonpain symptoms, quality of life, and mood has been largely, if not uniformly, confirmed by the results of the studies to date. Although not a defined palliative care domain, there has been significant interest in the impact of palliative care on resource use, particularly at end of life (eg, intensive care unit admissions, emergency department visits, hospice enrollment). The interest in this area stems from a desire to ensure that patient preferences for care are elicited and respected, particularly in patients at the most advanced stage of cancer when the burden of further cancer-directed therapy is likely highest and the benefits in terms of symptoms, quality of life, and mood are likely to be lowest. Integrated palliative care has been shown to enhance communication between patients and their providers about end-of-life preferences in patients with newly diagnosed lung and noncolorectal gastrointestinal cancers.[34] Patients with clear understanding of their prognoses who are able to articulate their preferences are more likely to receive care that matches their preferences (eg, intensive care, life support, symptom-focused care).[40] In addition, when patients with advanced cancer were able to discuss their wishes for end-of-life care with their physicians, they were less likely to receive mechanical ventilation, resuscitation, and intensive care unit admission compared with patients who did not have these discussions.[41] Importantly, these discussions were not associated with higher rates of major depressive disorder.

Table 2 summarizes the findings from 11 trials that examined the impact of a palliative care intervention on health care resource use. Three studies found that patients who received palliative care were more likely to die at home or in a nonacute facility,[42,45,46] whereas 2 studies did not show a difference in place of death in patients who received palliative care.[32,37] Data on the impact of palliative care on either the number of hospitalizations or duration of hospitalizations are mixed; 3 studies found a decrease, whereas 6 showed no difference in hospitalizations. Similarly, palliative care had a variable impact on hospice use; 3 studies did not show a difference in hospice use,[30,31,37] whereas another study did show an increase in hospice enrollment.[32] The timing of palliative care intervention has not been shown to affect resource use. A recent randomized controlled trial of patients who received palliative care early (on study enrollment) versus delayed (after 3 months) did not differ in any of the domains of resource use, including hospital days, intensive care unit days, or emergency department visits.[29]

Lastly, a limited number of studies have examined the impact of palliative care integration on survival. This area of investigation likely resulted from concerns that palliative care would result in reduced survival as patients and/or their caregivers elected for symptom-focused care rather than cancer-directed care. The landmark article by Temel and colleagues[19] found a 2.7-month increase in median survival with concurrent palliative care and standard cancer care in patients with metastatic NSCLC. In contrast, 1 year before this study was published, a randomized controlled trial by Bakitas and colleagues[25] did not find a difference in survival between the palliative care intervention and standard care groups. Interestingly, a follow-up study by the same group of early versus delayed palliative care found a 15% increase in 1-year survival in the group who received early palliative care compared with those who received palliative care 3 months later.[29] Two additional studies failed to show an improvement in survival with palliative care,[32,33] whereas 1 additional study did report a statistically nonsignificant doubling in median survival (132 days in the control group vs 289 days) in the palliative care intervention group.[31] Interpretation of the impact of integrated palliative care on survival is limited by numerous variables, including the setting in which palliative care is provided (outpatient vs inpatient) and estimated life expectancy based on tumor-related factors.

BARRIERS TO INTEGRATION OF PALLIATIVE CARE

Although much progress has been made toward earlier integration of palliative care into routine oncology care, significant barriers remain. A recent comprehensive overview on the integration of oncology and palliative care was published by the Lancet Oncology Commission.[47] In this overview, the investigators outline several barriers to integrating palliative care into oncology. They specifically mention the common misperception that palliative care is synonymous with end-of-life care, lack of perceived need by oncology providers for palliative care as an integral part of the cancer care continuum, inadequate access to palliative care specialists, lack of information regarding the cost and benefits of palliative care, and inadequate training by oncologists in primary palliative care. This last barrier highlights the need for competency in primary palliative care. In contrast with subspecialty palliative care, this refers to the ability of all cancer providers to have a basic proficiency in key palliative care domains.[48] The core competencies in surgical palliative care were outlined by Dr Geoffrey Dunn[49] in 2009. All surgeons are expected to be able to:

Table 2
Impact of palliative care on resource use

	Care Setting	Study Design	Location of Death	Hospitalization	Aggressiveness of Care	Hospice Use
Jordhøy et al,[42] 2000	Cooperation between palliative medicine unit and community service	N = 235 intervention N = 199 controls Cluster randomized trial	↑ Home	No difference	—	—
Costantini et al,[43] 2003	Palliative home care team	N = 189 PC, N = 378 control Quasiexperimental design	—	↓ Percentage of hospital days vs usual care	—	—
Miccinesi et al,[44] 2003	Home PC	N = 315 Retrospective review	—	↓ Hospitalizations ↓ days	—	—
Back et al,[45] 2005	PC service through Veterans' Administration	N = 82 PC N = 183 no PC Retrospective nonrandomized	↓ Death in acute care setting	—	↑ Chemotherapy in last 60 d of life	—
Bakitas et al,[25] 2009	Telephone sessions	N = 161 intervention N = 161 usual care RCT	—	No difference in # of hospital days, ICU admissions, or emergency department visits	—	—
Bakitas et al,[29] 2015	PC telehealth	N = 307 Random assignment of early vs late PC	No difference	No difference in hospital days, ICU days, emergency room visits	No difference in chemotherapy in last 14 d of life	—
Ferrell et al,[30] 2015	Outpatient PC	N = 491 Prospective, serial accrual of usual care followed by intervention group	—	No difference in unscheduled admissions	No difference in chemotherapy in the last 2 wk of life	No difference in hospice referral

(continued on next page)

Table 2
(continued)

	Care Setting	Study Design	Location of Death	Hospitalization	Aggressiveness of Care	Hospice Use
Grudzen et al,[31] 2016	Inpatient PC after emergency department referral	N = 69 PC N = 67 usual care RCT	—	No difference in hospital or ICU days	↓ Chemotherapy in the last 30 of life	No difference hospice enrollment
Maltoni et al,[32] 2016	Outpatient PC	N = 107 systematic PC N = 107 on demand PC Multicenter randomized trial	No difference	No difference in hospitalizations or emergency department visits	↓ Chemotherapy at end of life	↑ hospice use
Merchant et al,[46] 2018	Receipt of any PC services within 2 y of death	N = 24,241 received PC N = 10,389 no PC Retrospective analysis	↓ In-hospital death	↓ Hospitalization, ICU admissions, and emergency department visits	↓ Chemotherapy in last 30 d of life	—
Vanbutsele et al,[37] 2020	Outpatient PC	N = 91 integrated PC N = 94 usual care Random assignment	No difference	No difference	No difference in chemotherapy in last 30 d of life	No difference

Abbreviation: ICU, intensive care unit.

- Assess and treat pain and other symptoms
- Communicate effectively and compassionately bad news and poor prognoses
- Conduct a patient and family meeting regarding advanced directives and end-of-life decisions
- Perform palliative procedures competently and with sound judgment to meet patient goals of care
- Exercise sound clinical judgment and skill in the withdrawal and withholding of life support

Breaking down these remaining barriers to palliative care integration will depend on ongoing educational and research efforts. Some of the current guidelines for integrating palliative care into routine cancer care were formulated without the benefit of rigorous research, in contrast with the clinical trials routinely performed in other aspects of cancer care. Although National Institutes of Health (NIH) funding for palliative medicine investigators and the proportion of palliative medicine research funded by the NIH has increased in recent years, grants related to palliative care represented only 0.2% of all NIH research awards during the most recent time period studied.[50]

In addition to the barriers to integrating palliative care noted earlier, there exist unique challenges for surgical oncology patients. Suwanabol and colleagues[51] recently studied surgeon-perceived barriers to palliative care in patients with stage IV colorectal cancer. They reported that 76% of respondents had received no formal education in palliative care, highlighting the need for specific training in primary palliative care competencies. Surgeons also noted communication, difficulty in prognostication, and systemic issues related to culture and lack of appropriate resources as additional barriers to palliative care integration. The absence of expressed guidelines for integrating palliative care into surgical oncology by national surgical societies and lack of surgeon representation on expert panels tasked with providing guidelines on palliative care in oncology further hinder effective provision of palliative care services to surgical oncology patients.

SUMMARY AND RECOMMENDATIONS

Palliative care is now recognized as an essential component of cancer care. The road to this point has included several significant challenges, including an understanding of the distinction between palliative care and hospice and a lack of high-quality studies and clinical trials showing the beneficial effects of integrated palliative care. Although these challenges have been significantly addressed, several key questions remain: (1) what is the optimal model of delivery? (2) When is the ideal time to refer? (3) Which patients are in greatest need of a referral? (4) How much palliative care should oncologists themselves be providing?

While data from future studies that will address these questions are awaited, the following recommendations regarding integrated palliative care are appropriate for all oncology providers:

- All patients should be screened for palliative care needs at the time of diagnosis and at regular intervals
- Providers are expected to be able to provide primary palliative care
- Referral to subspecialty palliative medical providers should be provided for complex symptom management, severe emotional or psychosocial distress, spiritual or existential crisis, assistance with complex medical decision making, and on patient or caregiver request

- Education regarding the benefits of integrated palliative care with routine oncology care should be a component of training programs for all oncology providers

Given the unique issues associated with palliative surgical interventions (eg, procedural morbidity and mortality, impact of postoperative recovery on future cancer treatment), surgical societies that specialize in the care of patients with cancer are strongly advised to develop surgery-specific guidelines for integrating palliative care into routine surgical oncology care. Potential integration models may be needs based, prognosis based, or trigger based. A needs-based model would result in palliative care subspecialty consultation for patients with complex or difficult symptoms or needs. Prognosis-based palliative care referral is considered for patients with limited life expectancy, incurable cancer, and/or those with progressive disease despite treatment. Trigger-based palliative care relies on defined criteria to initiate palliative care consultation; these criteria typically use disease-based and prognosis-based triggers for referral, plus screening of unmet needs. The specific model used for integrating palliative care is likely to vary depending on unique characteristics of the population of patients with cancer, access to subspecialty palliative care services, and institutional resources. Regardless of the model used, oncology providers must commit to ensuring the palliative care services are available to their patients from diagnosis through end of life. Quality cancer care requires access and administration of palliative care concurrent with standard cancer care.

CLINICS CARE POINTS

- All patients with cancer, particularly those with advanced cancer, should be screened for palliative care needs at the time of diagnosis and throughout the course of cancer treatment, as well as when cancer-directed therapies are no longer provided.

- Palliative care should not be reserved for end-of-life care only.

- Cancer providers need to be aware of the pain and nonpain symptoms commonly experienced by patients with cancer and develop the knowledge and skills needed to address these needs through development of primary palliative care competency.

- Patients and their family members should be referred for subspecialty palliative care for complex symptom management, severe emotional or psychosocial distress, spiritual or existential crisis, assistance with complex medical decision making, and on patient or caregiver request.

DISCLOSURE

The author has no relevant financial interests to disclose.

REFERENCES

1. World Health Organization. Palliative care key facts. Available at: https://www.who.int/news-room/fact-sheets/detail/palliative-care. Accessed September 26, 2020.
2. National Consensus Project for Quality Palliative Care. Clinical practice guidelines for quality palliative care. 4th edition. Richmond (VA): National Coalition for Hospice and Palliative Care; 2018. Available at: https://www.nationalcoalitionhpc.org/ncp.

3. American Society of Clinical Oncology. Cancer care during the last phase of life. J Clin Oncol 1998;16:1986–96.
4. Ferris FD, Bruera E, Cherny N, et al. Palliative cancer care a decade later: accomplishments, the need, next steps—From the American Society of Clinical Oncology. J Clin Oncol 2009;27:3052–8.
5. Smith TJ, Temin S, Alesi ER, et al. American Society of Clinical Oncology provisional clinical opinion: the integration of palliative care into standard oncology care. J Clin Oncol 2012;30:880–7.
6. Ferrell BR, Temel JS, Temin S, et al. Integration of palliative care into standard oncology care: American Society of Clinical Oncology clinical practice guideline update. J Clin Oncol 2017;35:96–112.
7. Edwards MJ. Access to quality cancer care: consensus statement of the American Federation of Clinical Oncologic Societies. Ann Surg Oncol 1998;5:657–9.
8. Badgwell B. Will palliative care ever be cool? Ann Surg Oncol 2018;25:1799–800.
9. Field MJ, Cassel CK, editors. Institute of medicine: approaching death: improving care at the end of life. Washington, DC: National Academies Press; 1997.
10. Hewitt ME, Simone JV, National Cancer Policy Board (U.S.), editors. Ensuring quality cancer care. Washington, DC: National Academy Press; 1999.
11. National Research Council. Improving palliative care for cancer: summary and recommendations. Washington, DC: The National Academies Press; 2001.
12. National Academies of Sciences. Engineering and Medicine. Available at: https://www.nap.edu. Accessed September 26, 2020.
13. Commission on Cancer. cancer program standards 2012: ensuring patient-centered care. Available at: https://www.facs.org/~/media/files/quality%20programs/cancer/coc/programstandards2012.ashx. Accessed September 26, 2020.
14. Commission on Cancer. Cancer program standards 2016: ensuring patient-centered care. Available at: https://www.facs.org/~/media/files/quality%20programs/cancer/coc/2016%20coc%20standards%20manual_interactive%20pdf.ashx. Accessed September 26, 2020.
15. Commission on Cancer. Cancer program standards 2020: optimal resources for cancer care. Available at: https://www.facs.org/-/media/files/quality-programs/cancer/coc/optimal_resources_for_cancer_care_2020_standards.ashx. Accessed September 26, 2020.
16. National Comprehensive Cancer Network. Palliative care clinical practice guidelines in oncology. J Natl Compr Canc Netw 2003;1:394.
17. National Comprehensive Cancer Network. Palliative care clinical practice guidelines in oncology. Available at: https://www.nccn.org/professionals/physician_gls/pdf/palliative.pdf. Accessed September 26, 2020.
18. Higginson I, McCarthy M. Measuring symptoms in terminal cancer: are pain and dyspnoea controlled? J R Soc Med 1989;82:264–7.
19. Temel JS, Greer JA, Muzikansky A, et al. Early palliative care for patients with metastatic non-small-cell lung cancer. N Engl J Med 2010;363:733–42.
20. Ellershaw JE, Peat SJ, Boys LC. Assessing the effectiveness of a hospital palliative care team. Palliat Med 1995;9:145–52.
21. Peruselli C, Paci E, Franceschi P, et al. Outcome evaluation in a home palliative care service. J Pain Symptom Manage 1997;13:158–65.
22. Mercadante S, Fulfaro F, Casuccio A. The impact of home palliative care on symptoms in advanced cancer patients. Support Care Cancer 2000;8:307–10.
23. Jordhøy MS, Fayers P, Loge JH, et al. Quality of life in palliative cancer care: results from a cluster randomized trial. J Clin Oncol 2001;19:3884–94.

24. Strömgren AS, Sjogren P, Goldschmidt D, et al. A longitudinal study of palliative care: patient-evaluated outcome and impact of attrition. Cancer 2005;103: 1747–55.

25. Bakitas M, Lyons KD, Hegel MT, et al. Effects of a palliative care intervention on clinical outcomes in patients with advanced cancer: the Project ENABLE II randomized controlled trial. JAMA 2009;302:741–9.

26. Follwell M, Burman D, Le LW, et al. Phase II study of an outpatient palliative care intervention in patients with metastatic cancer. J Clin Oncol 2009;27:206–13.

27. Bischoff K, Weinberg V, Rabow MW. Palliative and oncologic co-management: symptom management for outpatients with cancer. Support Care Cancer 2013; 21:3031–7.

28. Zimmermann C, Swami N, Krzyzanowska M, et al. Early palliative care for patients with advanced cancer: a cluster-randomised controlled trial. Lancet 2014;383: 1721–30.

29. Bakitas MA, Tosteson TD, Li Z, et al. Early versus delayed initiation of concurrent palliative oncology care: patient outcomes in the ENABLE III randomized controlled trial. J Clin Oncol 2015;33:1438–45.

30. Ferrell B, Sun V, Hurria A, et al. Interdisciplinary palliative care for patients with lung cancer. J Pain Symptom Manage 2015;50:758–67.

31. Grudzen CR, Richardson LD, Johnson PN, et al. Emergency department-initiated palliative care in advanced cancer: a randomized clinical trial. JAMA Oncol 2016; 2:591–8.

32. Maltoni M, Scarpi E, Dall'Agata M, et al. Systematic versus on-demand early palliative care: results from a multicentre, randomised clinical trial. Eur J Cancer 2016; 65:61–8.

33. Groenvold M, Petersen MA, Damkier A, et al. Randomised clinical trial of early specialist palliative care plus standard care versus standard care alone in patients with advanced cancer: The Danish Palliative Care Trial. Palliat Med 2017; 31:814–24.

34. Temel JS, Greer JA, El-Jawahri A, et al. Effects of early integrated palliative care in patients with lung and GI cancer: a randomized clinical trial. J Clin Oncol 2017; 35:834–41.

35. Johnsen AT, Petersen MA, Sjøgren P, et al. Exploratory analyses of the Danish Palliative Care Trial (DanPaCT): a randomized trial of early specialized palliative care plus standard care versus standard care in advanced cancer patients. Support Care Cancer 2020;28:2145–55.

36. Slama O, Pochop L, Sedo J, et al. Effects of early and systematic integration of specialist palliative care in patients with advanced cancer: randomized controlled trial PALINT. J Palliat Med 2020;23(12):1586–93.

37. Vanbutsele G, Van Belle S, Surmont V, et al. The effect of early and systematic integration of palliative care in oncology on quality of life and health care use near the end of life: a randomised controlled trial. Eur J Cancer 2020;124:186–93.

38. European Organisation for Research Treatment of Cancer. Quality of Life Cancer Patients. Available at: https://qol.eortc.org. Accessed September 26, 2020.

39. Peterman AH, Fitchett G, Brady MJ, et al. Measuring spiritual well-being in people with cancer: the functional assessment of chronic illness therapy–Spiritual Well-being Scale (FACIT-Sp). Ann Behav Med 2002;24:49–58.

40. Mack JW, Weeks JC, Wright AA, et al. End-of-life discussions, goal attainment, and distress at the end of life: predictors and outcomes of receipt of care consistent with preferences. J Clin Oncol 2010;28:1203–8.

41. Wright AA, Zhang B, Ray A, et al. Associations between end-of-life discussions, patient mental health, medical care near death, and caregiver bereavement adjustment. JAMA 2008;300:1665–73.
42. Jordhøy MS, Fayers P, Saltnes T, et al. A palliative-care intervention and death at home: a cluster randomised trial. Lancet 2000;356:888–93.
43. Costantini M, Higginson IJ, Boni L, et al. Effect of a palliative home care team on hospital admissions among patients with advanced cancer. Palliat Med 2003;17: 315–21.
44. Miccinesi G, Crocetti E, Morino P, et al. Palliative home care reduces time spent in hospital wards: a population-based study in the Tuscany Region, Italy. Cancer Causes Control 2003;14:971–7.
45. Back AL, Li Y-F, Sales AE. Impact of palliative care case management on resource use by patients dying of cancer at a Veterans Affairs medical center. J Palliat Med 2005;8:26–35.
46. Merchant SJ, Brogly SB, Goldie C, et al. Palliative care is associated with reduced aggressive end-of-life care in patients with gastrointestinal cancer. Ann Surg Oncol 2018;25:1478–87.
47. Kaasa S, Loge JH, Aapro M, et al. Integration of oncology and palliative care: a Lancet Oncology Commission. Lancet Oncol 2018;19:e588–653.
48. von Gunten CF. Secondary and tertiary palliative care in US hospitals. JAMA 2002;287:875–81.
49. Dunn GP. Principles and core competencies of surgical palliative care: an overview. Otolaryngol Clin North Am 2009;42:1–13.
50. Brown E, Morrison RS, Gelfman LP. An update: NIH research funding for palliative medicine, 2011-2015. J Palliat Med 2018;21:182–7.
51. Suwanabol PA, Reichstein AC, Suzer-Gurtekin ZT, et al. Surgeons' perceived barriers to palliative and end-of-life care: a mixed methods study of a surgical society. J Palliat Med 2018;21:780–8.

Selecting Patients for Palliative Procedures in Oncology

Cassandra S. Parker, MD, Thomas J. Miner, MD*

KEYWORDS

• Palliative surgery • Palliative triangle • Oncology • Patient selection

KEY POINTS

- Patient selection for palliative procedures is one of the most important determinants of benefit.
- Clear communication between the patient, patient family, and the surgeon via the *palliative triangle* is imperative in appropriately selecting patients for palliative interventions.
- Appropriate patient selection takes into account patient-specific factors, such as values, end-of-life priorities, symptom characteristics and life expectancy, as well as predictors of patient benefit and risk from a specific intervention.

INTRODUCTION

Almost 40% of the US population will be diagnosed with cancer during their lifetimes and over 600,000 people will die secondary to advanced cancer in the United States in 2020.[1] As patients present with or develop disease that is no longer amendable to curative therapy, it is the role of the physician to transition attempts to improve patient quality of life, rather than focusing on prolongation of life. This classification of medicine, termed "palliative care" by surgeon Dr Balfour Mount in 1975[2] has been defined by the World Health Organization as care that "improves the quality of life of patients and their families facing the problem associated with life-threatening illness, through prevention and relief of suffering by means of early identification and impeccable assessment and treatment of pain and other problems."[3]

Surgeons perform an essential role in palliative cancer care, as common complications of late-stage malignancy include diagnoses considered indications for operative intervention including gastric, bowel or biliary obstruction, gastric or bowel perforation, bleeding, and advanced wound management.[4–6] As such, the surgeon's role in end-of-life care has become an area of focus in surgical training, and after undergoing palliative care–specific training, residents have acknowledged the value of that

Department of Surgery, Rhode Island Hospital, Warren Alpert Medical School of Brown University, 593 Eddy Street, APC 443, Providence, RI 02903, USA
* Corresponding author.
E-mail address: TMiner@Lifespan.org

Surg Oncol Clin N Am 30 (2021) 449–459
https://doi.org/10.1016/j.soc.2021.02.006
1055-3207/21/© 2021 Elsevier Inc. All rights reserved.
surgonc.theclinics.com

training.[7] Bradley and colleagues even developed "core competencies in palliative care for surgeons" that focus on the development of necessary communication and empathy skills to facilitate palliative care discussions.[8] In addition, surgeon knowledge and involvement in palliative care has become a priority among leading societies, and the American College of Surgeons established the, "Principles Guiding Care at the End of Life" with such dictums as "ensure alleviation of pain and management of other physical symptoms," "provide access to therapies that may realistically be expected to improve the patient's quality of life," "respect the patient's right to refuse treatment," and "recognize the physician's responsibility to forego treatments that are futile."[9] Meeting these expectations is a balancing act that challenges even the most experienced surgeons, but is worth the effort, as providing appropriate relief of suffering to our patients in order to maximize quality of life at the end of their lives while not exposing them to undue morbidity or hastened mortality is a truly noble and necessary endeavor.

In comparison to palliative care provided by medical palliative care providers, surgical and procedural palliative care requires invasive intervention, which introduces increased risk for the patient, and therefore, the intervention itself requires special consideration. In comparison to curative-intent interventions, palliative operations are aimed at the alleviation of symptoms, rather than eradication of disease. Although not mutually exclusive, explicitly defining operative intent refines an operative plan to achieve the outcome of symptom relief without the additional risk that may be necessary for complete resection of disease[4,10]; this is exemplified by a study of noncurative gastric cancer resections that observed that patients whose cases were designated as being performed with palliative intent preoperatively underwent a significantly less extensive lymphadenectomy as well as less frequent esophageal anastomoses, indicating that identifying operative intent as palliative does lead to a meaningfully different intervention.[10] Therefore, surgical palliation may be defined as, "procedures employed with non-curative intent with the primary goal of improving symptoms caused by an advanced malignancy," as previously established by this author.[11]

Palliative operations can lead to substantial symptom relief in patients with end-stage malignancies but can also be wrought with high morbidity and mortality.[4,11–13] For instance, a series of 1022 palliative procedures performed at a high-volume cancer center found that intervention resulted in symptom improvement 80% of the time, but with 29% morbidity and 11% mortality within 30 days.[11] Another study with 240 palliative procedures showed similar results with morbidity of 21.3% and mortality of 12.3% within 30 days.[12] This increased risk of complications often results in prolonged inpatient hospitalization, additional interventions, additional or worsened symptoms, and hastened death, ultimately resulting in further patient suffering and decreased quality of life at the end of life. Therefore, appropriate patient and procedure selection is imperative in order to maximize patient benefit while minimizing risk.

OPERATIVE PALLIATION CANDIDATE SELECTION

The first step in the evaluation of a patient presenting with an advanced and noncurable malignancy seeking symptom alleviation is to assess the indication for intervention, which requires a thorough and specific definition of the problem that the patient is presenting with, including the nature, extent and severity of symptoms, projected disease trajectory and life expectancy, patient values and goals for end-of-life care, and what risks or tradeoffs they are willing to accept to attain specific goals.[4,5,14]

Interventions performed with curative intent have well-defined risks of treatment toxicity, complications, and rare mortality, which are tolerated, as the intent of the intervention is disease cure, which offers sufficient potential benefit to render the risks acceptable. In contrast, the goal of an oncologic palliative intervention is to improve the quality of life or reduce symptoms in a patient with an advanced malignancy. Given that treatment toxicity or complications will adversely affect the ability to obtain these palliative goals, and may result in increased suffering, it is necessary that potential treatment toxicity and morbidity be outweighed by likely symptom alleviation.[4,5,14]

Determining the suitability of a palliative intervention for a given patient is a complex process that requires an in-depth understanding of that patient's disease process, as well as his or her priorities and goals of care. Any intervention comes with trade-offs — offering the possibility of relief from a set of current symptoms but with the risk of creating new or worsened issues. It is therefore crucial that a clinician appreciate not only the quality and severity of a patient's symptoms but also his or her values and how he or she prioritizes various, commonly competing end-of-life outcomes. For instance, minimization of pain may result in increased somnolence and decreased quality time spent with loved ones, or an operative intervention may relieve a bowel obstruction and allow for oral intake, but result in postoperative pain or complications requiring increased hospitalization. Understanding what value a patient places on these outcomes is imperative to perform an appropriate risk/benefit analysis.[4,6,15]

In addition to an appreciation of a patient's symptoms and end-of-life priorities, consideration of the current extent of disease, likely progression of disease, and estimated life expectancy is necessary. Extent of disease may affect the feasibility of a given intervention effectively alleviating symptoms. For instance, small bowel obstruction secondary to disseminated metastasis is much less likely to be amendable to operative bypass than a focal obstruction from the primary tumor site and therefore will likely require proximal stoma creation, which should be established and communicated with the patient before intervention.[16,17] It is also important to consider projected life expectancy when choosing among various palliative interventions that may offer different recovery times with the trade-off of durability. For instance, No and colleagues examined outcomes in patients with gastric outlet obstruction secondary to inoperable gastric cancer following treatment with either self-expanding metal stents or surgical gastrojejunostomy and found that patients with good functional status experienced more prolonged relief of obstruction (282 vs 125 days) with fewer requirements for reintervention after undergoing operative intervention than stenting. Therefore, if a patient has a life expectancy of longer than the expected patency of the stent and can physiologically tolerate an operative intervention, gastrojejunostomy would be preferred over endoscopic stenting.[18]

Careful communication with a patient about symptoms, priorities in end-of-life care, extent of disease, and expected disease progression will allow the physician to provide a comprehensive but also targeted explanation of what outcomes are possible from a given intervention, including the degree and durability of symptom relief, as well as costs or trade-offs associated with the intervention.[4,6,15] An effective methodology to facilitate this communication is the *palliative triangle*, which is a process of shared decision-making between the patient, the patient's family, and the attending surgeon. Through this methodology, each party first defines a specific problem to be addressed and ensures that there is agreement on the details of this problem. Once the problem is clearly identified, the patient and patient's support system provide information regarding symptom severity, personal values, and end-of-life priorities. The surgeon then discusses any available palliative interventions, including details regarding risks, expected durability, and availability of other modalities to alleviate symptoms. Finally, the group discusses how all of these pieces fit together — given the patient's current extent of disease and life expectancy, what intervention, if any, is likely to result in maximal achievement of that patient's end-of-life priorities, while minimizing unacceptable risks. This discussion allows the entire group to then arrive at a shared decision. The *palliative triangle* has been shown to improve patient selection and patient perception of success after palliative interventions.[6,11,15] Miner and colleagues found that when evaluating a patient for a palliative procedure, using the *palliative triangle* frequently leads to a decision by the patient not to undergo the intervention, with 23.9% due to low severity of symptoms, 19.8% due to patient preference, and 19% because nonoperative palliation was selected.[15] Furthermore, of the patients who did undergo interventional palliation, 90% reported symptom improvement or resolution versus 80% in a large study that was performed around the same time and with otherwise similar patient selection standards.[11]

In addition, in 2014 Blakely and colleagues showed that 88% of patients who underwent a palliative operation for advanced cancer symptoms expressed the feeling that the intervention was "worth it," despite the fact that 18% of these patients did not experience any symptom relief after intervention. This study was performed at a hospital where the palliative triangle was used in thorough preoperative patient education and was thought by the investigators to be the likely cause for this phenomenon.[19] Although the *palliative triangle* focuses on the participation of the attending surgeon in discussions with the patient and his or her family, other groups have emphasized the importance of nursing involvement in these end-of-life discussions in hospitalized patients, especially for those in the intensive care unit (ICU).[17] Nurses in the ICU regularly care for patients with advanced disease states, are trained to identify potentially overlooked symptoms, and commonly form close relationships with patients and their families. Therefore, they are in a unique position to assist in bridging any gaps in communication between physicians and the patient and his or her family and play an important role in palliative care discussions for patients in the ICU.[20,21]

Exemplifying the growing focus on shared decision-making in palliative decisions, an interdisciplinary panel of 23 national leaders involved in emergency operations in elderly and frail patients met in 2014. Nine key elements of "best communication practices" were identified that included a focus on early prognosis formulation, followed by creating a personal connection and elicitation of the patient and his or her family's priorities and goals, and a full disclosure of the patient's illness and available palliative interventions. They then recommend integrating information obtained from the patient with provider-knowledge in order to offer a treatment recommendation, while allowing for silence, acknowledging and dealing with emotions, and continuing to check back in with the patient and family in order to confirm ongoing buy-in and support with the established decisions.[22] Although preoperative communication is essential, it is also imperative to have repeated communication any time that a patient's expected trajectory changes, such as after a complication or on unexpected disease progression. Schwarze and colleagues discussed surgeon bias and demonstrated through the use of a survey that most of the surgeons believe that by agreeing to an operation, patients are also agreeing to continue to undergo life-saving measures for a period of time postoperatively, although this is not explicitly stated in the consent process.[23,24] It is therefore essential that we actively revisit goals of care throughout a patient's postoperative course to ensure that we, as surgeons, are not mistaking our own biases for the wishes of the patient.

Another factor that affects selection of appropriate candidates for palliative intervention is the patient's anticipated life expectancy. Given that the goal of palliative care is to improve quality of life, rather than the duration of life, when considering palliative interventions, the use of overall survival as a primary outcome is inappropriate, but this information can give useful context to the palliative decision-making process.

Life expectancy can be particularly important when considering a patient for a particular intervention in relation to its benefit and risk profile.[4] Procedures with more durable palliation may come with a higher up-front risk of morbidity. For instance, a systematic review that examined stenting versus surgery in patients with malignant large bowel obstruction found that although short-term complication rates were similar, patients who underwent stent placement experienced a quicker recovery, allowing for a shorter length of hospital stay, but also experienced increased late complications such as stent migration, requiring stent replacement, as well as a 2-fold increased incidence of bowel perforation.[25] Therefore, in a patient with very limited life expectancy, it may be appropriate to recommend endoscopic stenting, allowing for the minimalization of short-term morbidity with a less invasive procedure, while still avoiding late complications or the necessity of a reintervention due to decreased durability of the procedure, given the patient's limited life expectancy. In contrast, a patient with a longer life expectancy may opt for operative intervention in order to have a lower risk of late complications and a more durable intervention, potentially avoiding the need for repeat intervention.[5]

It may then become important for a surgeon to be able to predict patient survival in order to better recommend the appropriate therapy. There are many available prognostic tools available, and a recent systematic review examined 7 of them over 49 studies.[26] The investigators found that the Glasgow Prognostic Score (GPS)[27] was the most favorable due to its ease to administer and use of only 2 parameters, both of which are objective measures of inflammation and malnutrition. In addition, they felt that it was beneficial that GPS does not include less objective instruments, such as performance status, as they can be used along-side one another to provide a more complete prognostic picture while not blurring the lines between physiologic markers provided by GPS and functional measures, such as performance status.[26,27]

BENEFITS OF PALLIATIVE OPERATIONS

As with all interventions, it is necessary to establish the therapeutic index (benefits vs risks or costs) of a given palliative operation in order to determine if the intervention is likely to provide patient benefit in excess of potential risks incurred. Defining benefit of a palliative intervention is complex, as traditional oncologic and surgical measures such as tumor remission and disease-free or overall survival are not the primary goals of palliative procedures. Although relief of symptoms and improved quality of life is defined differently by each patient, various methods have been used to measure benefits after a palliative procedure, including changes in quality of life,[28] patient-reported symptom improvement,[5,11–13] and patient-reported satisfaction with the procedure.[5,19,29]

Symptom Improvement

There are several ways to gauge patient benefit after a palliative intervention, and one of the most common is to assess for alleviation of symptoms. One study examined symptom improvement or resolution in patients with advanced malignancy who received a consultation for a palliative operation, regardless of whether or not the patient underwent the operation. They found that out of 202 consultations, 17% underwent a palliative procedure, 43% a palliative operation, and 40% were managed medically. Notably, almost 70% of patients experienced symptoms improvement, which includes 60% of those managed medically, 69% of those who underwent a procedure, and 78% of those operatively managed. The definition for symptom improvement varied based on patient presentation, but for instance, resolution of bowel obstruction, which was the most common reason for consultation, was defined as the ability to tolerate an oral diet without the need for parenteral nutrition, and resolution of wound issues, as the second most common reason for evaluation, was defined as improved signs of skin or soft tissue infection, reported improvement in pain, and decreased wound drainage.[30]

Another valuable way to evaluate the benefit of a palliative intervention is through patient-reported symptom improvement or resolution. This method has been used in several studies and has shown that in carefully selected patient populations, 75% to 80% reported an improvement or resolution of symptoms. Unfortunately, these studies also showed that 16% to 25% patients experienced recurrence of symptoms and 23% to 29% developed new symptoms.[5,11,13] Therefore, although most patients were able to achieve benefit, it was with limited durability, and therefore overall benefit may be overestimated without considering duration of benefit. As discussed previously, it is essential to consider the trade-off between immediate morbidity, which can be minimized with less invasive procedures such as stents for large bowel obstruction[17,31] or gastric outlet obstruction,[18] and durability, which may be maximized with a more invasive operative intervention, with a reduced likely need for reintervention for those patients with a longer life expectancy.[17,18,31] Of note, a separate study examining outcomes in patients with malignant bowel obstruction secondary to peritoneal carcinomatosis after a palliative operation found that 35% of the patients experienced repeat obstruction.[32] Therefore, it is necessary to consider not only the durability of the intervention but also the predicted trajectory of a given disease state when determining whether symptom improvement is an appropriate descriptor of patient benefit.

A potential limitation of using symptom improvement as the sole determinant of patient benefit from a palliative intervention is that it may be too narrow in scope—missing other benefits that the patient may derive from an intervention. For instance, a series of 26 patients who underwent palliative oncologic interventions showed that although only 46% showed symptom improvement, patients reported a significant improvement in physical and functional well-being on 30-day postprocedural surveys.[13] These data suggest that the patients derive benefits from the operation other than symptomatic improvement. From this perspective, symptom resolution may be appropriate to determine overall clinical success of the intervention but may be inadequate to capture overall patient benefit.

Overall Patient Satisfaction

An alternative and potentially more comprehensive way to assess the efficacy of a palliative intervention is to ask the patient whether or not the intervention was "worth it." This methodology was applied in 2 studies by the same investigators—one examining predictors of success in palliative cancer operations[29] and the other evaluating efficacy of palliative interventions for locoregional control in soft tissue and metastatic malignancies.[19] In both studies more patients stated that the intervention was "worth it" than experienced objective symptom improvement. This simple method is able to account for all subjective differences in how patients interpret the impact of the intervention on the quality of their lives and capture any trade-off due to short duration of benefit or complications from the intervention, includes unforeseen benefits that the patient may derive from the intervention, and therefore is likely the most comprehensive and easily applied evaluation of efficacy of a palliative intervention.[5,19,29]

RISKS OF PALLIATIVE CARE OPERATIONS

Determining the risk of palliative operations requires consideration of patient, procedure, and disease-related factors. The high rates of morbidity (40%) and mortality (11%)

following palliative procedure has been well established.[11] One series observed 30-day mortality of 31% but noted that half of the deceased patients did so from progression of disease.[13] In addition, palliative care patients are known to be at higher risk for complications as compared with the general population.[4,5,14]

There are numerous methods available to estimate risk for patients undergoing palliative oncologic interventions. Most of them include some measures of preoperative functional status, nutritional status, comorbidities, and overall physiologic status (immune dysregulation, anemia, etc.).[5] Functional status is frequently measured by scales such as the Eastern Cooperative Oncology Group (ECOG) Scale of Performance measure or the National Cancer Institute (NCI) fatigue score. The former grades a patient from zero (fully functional) to five (dead) based on ability to perform work and self-care, ambulate, and spend time out of bed during waking hours,[33] and the latter is simply a subjective score with zero as normal levels of fatigue and higher numbers indicating increasing levels of fatigue.[34] Nutritional status is commonly derived either by using proxies, such as recent unintentional weight loss or serum albumin levels, or by indices such as the Prognostic Nutritional Index.[35] Comorbidity burden may be based on formal classifications, such as the American Society of Anesthesiologists physical status classification or by correlating with individual comorbidities. Attempts to capture other forms of physiologic dysfunction can be based on low hemoglobin levels, irregular white blood cell (WBC) counts, or other markers of inflammation dysregulation such as C-reactive protein (CRP) levels. Most clinicians tend to use a mixture of these markers, and there are several formal indices that combine these in an attempt to predict palliative operative risk. Here the authors review some of the evidence behind different methods used.[36]

One recent study used ability to rise from a chair as a proxy for functional status and was able to show that this independently predicted top quartile survival among 167 patients who underwent oncologic operations with a palliative intent at a single institution.[37] A prospective review of 823 patients who underwent 1022 palliative procedures found that reduced survival was associated with decreased functional status—defined as ECOG greater than or equal to 2 and/or NCI fatigue score greater than or equal to 1; poor nutritional status—defined as albumin less than 3.5 or significant weight loss of greater than or equal to $\geq$10 pounds in the past 90 days; and lack of prior cancer therapy. Of these factors, albumin less than 3.5 and ECOG greater than or equal to $\geq$2 were only found to be significant on multivariate analysis.[11] Other investigators found that major complications and decreased survival correlated with CRP levels and an NCI fatigue score greater than or equal to 1 on univariate analysis but only CRP levels on multivariate analysis.[29] In contrast, they did not find an association between ECOG scale, low albumin, significant weight loss, or prior cancer therapy and survival.[29] Another retrospective review of 37 patients with advanced colorectal adenocarcinoma who underwent operative palliation found that morbidity correlated with a lower Prognostic Nutritional Index—a value based on hypoalbuminemia and lymphopenia—as well as the presence of ascites.[38]

Other studies that have examined surgical risk in patients with cancer undergoing urgent or emergent abdominal operations, not specifically palliative, include the study by Roses and colleagues.[39] They found that ASA was greater than 3 and creatinine greater than 1.3, the operation being performed for a tumor-related indication (vs appendicitis or cholecystitis, for example), and the presence of active disease were independent predictors of decreased overall survival. They suggest the use of a "palliative index" to predict outcomes following emergent operations in patients with cancer, with more weight given to the presence of active disease. Of note, this study included patients with active and nonactive malignancies, such that less than 50%

had stage IV disease, and many of the operations were not palliative in nature, which may limit the applicability of this index to palliative procedures.[39]

A study by Tseng and colleagues used data from the American College of Surgeons National Surgical Quality Improvement Program (ACS NSQIP) to create a nomogram to predict 30-day morbidity and mortality in patients with disseminated malignancy who require and operative intervention.[40] They reviewed 7447 cases and found the following variables were independently associated with increased morbidity and mortality: code status of do-not-resuscitate, weight loss greater than 10% in past 6 months, chronic steroid use, active sepsis, elevated creatinine, hypoalbuminemia, abnormal WBC, anemia, higher acuity procedures, and more invasive procedure types (multivisceral > appendectomy or cholecystectomy > vascular > soft tissue). They created a nomogram that assigns a risk score for 30-day morbidity and mortality with concordance indices of 0.704 and 0.861, respectively.[40] Although this may be useful as a tool for predicting risk in all patients with disseminated cancer undergoing an operation, it may not be applicable to patients undergoing palliative operations, specifically. A study by Vidri and colleagues also used the ACS NSQIP database to study for patients with advanced cancer undergoing surgical procedures.[41] They attempted to compare outcomes in operations with and without palliative intent and found no difference in 30-day mortality. The investigators then did a chart review within their institutional electronic medical record of patients who underwent palliative procedures and were able to find that overall survival was significantly lower in operations with a palliative intent (104 vs 709 days). This study suggests that information in NSQIP is not comprehensive enough to appropriately designate operations as palliative in nature, and therefore is insufficient to predict outcomes for patients undergoing palliative operations.[41] Another study examined the ability of the American College of Surgeons Risk Calculator (ACSRC) to accurately predict patient length of stay (LOS) and risk for postoperative complications in patients with advanced cancer undergoing palliative procedures. They queried a prospectively maintained surgical oncology database for patients who underwent palliative procedures over a 2-year period and compared rates of complications and LOS from the medical record with those that would be predicted using the ACSRC and found that it overestimated the likelihood of postoperative complications and underestimated patient LOS. This tool may therefore not be wholly applicable in the palliative oncologic population and therefore should be used with caution in predicting patient outcomes.[42]

SUMMARY

Surgeons are important providers of palliative procedures—those performed with noncurative intent in order to relieve symptoms or improve quality of life in patients with incurable disease. Although palliative procedures in patients with advanced and incurable malignancies can provide very meaningful benefits, they come with a higher rate of morbidity and mortality than nonpalliative interventions. These risks can be minimized with careful patient selection, which should be based on the patient's indication for intervention including symptom characteristics, patient priorities, and values, disease trajectory and life expectancy, as well as predicted patient benefit and risks. Appropriate determination of the patient's indication within the framework of their personal values as well as the likelihood that he or she will achieve benefit is best achieved by open communication via the palliative triangle method with the patient, the patient's family, and the surgeon. Assessing patient risks is difficult but is likely best achieved by looking at their overall physiologic picture including functional status, nutritional status, and any signs of organ dysfunction or immune dysregulation. Lastly, assessing whether the patient benefited from the palliative intervention can be done via a simple measure that allows the patient to reflect on all potential benefits against any harms from the intervention, such as asking if the intervention was "worth it."

DISCLOSURE

None.

REFERENCES

1. Cancer of Any Site - Cancer Stat Facts. SEER. 2020. Available at: https://seer. cancer.gov/statfacts/html/all.html. Accessed September 7, 2020.
2. Duffy A. A moral force: the story of Dr. Balfour Mount The Ottawa Citizen; 2005.
3. Sepúlveda C, Marlin A, Yoshida T, et al. Palliative care: the World Health Organization's global perspective. J Pain Symptom Manag 2002;24(2):91–6.
4. Miner TJ. Palliative surgery for advanced cancer: lessons learned in patient selection and outcome assessment. Am J Clin Oncol 2005;28(4):411–4.
5. Cohen JT, Miner TJ. Patient selection in palliative surgery: Defining value. J Surg Oncol 2019;120(1):35–44.
6. Thomay AA, Jaques DP, Miner TJ. Surgical palliation: getting back to our roots. Surg Clin North Am 2009;89(1):27–41.
7. Klaristenfeld DD, Harrington DT, Miner TJ. Teaching palliative care and end-of-life issues: a core curriculum for surgical residents. Ann Surg Oncol 2007;14(6):1801.
8. Bradley CT, Brasel KJ. Core competencies in palliative care for surgeons: interpersonal and communication skills. Am J Hosp Palliat Med 2008;24(6):499–507.
9. American College of Surgeons' Committee on Ethics Statement on principles guiding care at the end of life. Bull Am Coll Surg 1998;83(4):46.
10. Miner TJ, Jaques DP, Karpeh MS, et al. Defining palliative surgery in patients receiving noncurative resections for gastric cancer. J Am Coll Surg 2004; 198(6):1013–21.
11. Miner TJ, Brennan MF, Jaques DP. A prospective, symptom related, outcomes analysis of 1022 palliative procedures for advanced cancer. Ann Surg 2004; 240(4):719.
12. Krouse RS, Nelson RA, Farrell BR, et al. Surgical palliation at a cancer center: incidence and outcomes. Arch Surg 2001;136(7):773–8.
13. Miner TJ, Jaques DP, Shriver CD. A prospective evaluation of patients undergoing surgery for the palliation of an advanced malignancy. Ann Surg Oncol 2002; 9(7):696–703.
14. Folkert IW, Roses RE. Value in palliative cancer surgery: a critical assessment. J Surg Oncol 2016;114(3):311–5.
15. Miner TJ, Cohen J, Charpentier K, et al. The palliative triangle: improved patient selection and outcomes associated with palliative operations. Arch Surg 2011; 146(5):517–23.
16. Drake TM, Lee MJ, Sayers AE, et al. Outcomes following small bowel obstruction due to malignancy in the national audit of small bowel obstruction. Eur J Surg Oncol 2019;45(12):2319–24.
17. Furnes B, Svensen R, Helland H, et al. Challenges and outcome of surgery for bowel obstruction in women with gynaecologic cancer. Int J Surg 2016;27: 158–64.
18. No JH, Kim SW, Lim C-H, et al. Long-term outcome of palliative therapy for gastric outlet obstruction caused by unresectable gastric cancer in patients with good

performance status: endoscopic stenting versus surgery. Gastrointest Endosc 2013;78(1):55–62.

19. Blakely AM, McPhillips J, Miner TJ. Surgical palliation for malignant disease requiring locoregional control. Ann Palliat Med 2015;4(2):48–53.

20. Nelson JE, Cortez TB, Curtis JR, et al. Integrating palliative care in the ICU: the nurse in a leading role. J Hosp Palliat Nurs 2011;13(2):89.

21. Fox MY. Improving communication with patients and families in the intensive care unit: palliative care strategies for the intensive care unit nurse. J Hosp Palliat Nurs 2014;16(2):93–8.

22. Cooper Z, Koritsanszky LA, Cauley CE, et al. Recommendations for best communication practices to facilitate goal-concordant care for seriously ill older patients with emergency surgical conditions. Ann Surg 2016;263(1):1–6.

23. Schwarze ML, Bradley CT, Brasel KJ. Surgical "buy-in": the contractual relationship between surgeons and patients that influences decisions regarding life-supporting therapy. Crit Care Med 2010;38(3):843.

24. Schwarze ML, Redmann AJ, Alexander GC, et al. Surgeons expect patients to buy-in to postoperative life support preoperatively: results of a national survey. Crit Care Med 2013;41(1):1.

25. Liang T-w, Sun Y, Wei Y-c, et al. Palliative treatment of malignant colorectal obstruction caused by advanced malignancy: a self-expanding metallic stent or surgery? A system review and meta-analysis. Surg Today 2014;44(1):22–33.

26. Simmons CP, McMillan DC, McWilliams K, et al. Prognostic tools in patients with advanced cancer: a systematic review. J Pain Symptom Manag 2017;53(5): 962–70.e10.

27. Nozoe T, Matono R, Ijichi H, et al. Glasgow Prognostic Score (GPS) can be a useful indicator to determine prognosis of patients with colorectal carcinoma. Int Surg 2014;99(5):512–7.

28. McCaffrey N, Bradley S, Ratcliffe J, et al. What aspects of quality of life are important from palliative care patients' perspectives? A systematic review of qualitative research. J Pain Symptom Manag 2016;52(2):318–28.e5.

29. Blakely AM, Heffernan DS, McPhillips J, et al. Elevated C-reactive protein as a predictor of patient outcomes following palliative surgery. J Surg Oncol 2014; 110(6):651–5.

30. Badgwell BD, Aloia TA, Garrett J, et al. Indicators of symptom improvement and survival in inpatients with advanced cancer undergoing palliative surgical consultation. J Surg Oncol 2013;107(4):367–71.

31. Siddiqui A, Cosgrove N, Yan LH, et al. Long-term outcomes of palliative colonic stenting versus emergency surgery for acute proximal malignant colonic obstruction: a multicenter trial. Endosc Int open 2017;5(4):E232.

32. de Boer NL, Hagemans JA, Schultze BT, et al. Acute malignant obstruction in patients with peritoneal carcinomatosis: the role of palliative surgery. Eur J Surg Oncol 2019;45(3):389–93.

33. Oken MM, Creech RH, Tormey DC, et al. Toxicity and response criteria of the Eastern Cooperative Oncology Group. Am J Clin Oncol 1982;5(6):649–56.

34. Berger AM, Mitchell SA, Jacobsen PB, et al. Screening, evaluation, and management of cancer-related fatigue: Ready for implementation to practice? CA Cancer J Clin 2015;65(3):190–211.

35. Sato R, Oikawa M, Kakita T, et al. The prognostic value of the prognostic nutritional index and inflammation-based markers in obstructive colorectal cancer. Surg Today 2020;50(10):1272–81.

36. Hui D. Prognostication of survival in patients with advanced cancer: predicting the unpredictable? Cancer Control 2015;22(4):489–97.
37. Cohen JT, Fallon EA, Charpentier KP, et al. Improving the value of palliative surgery by optimizing patient selection: The role of long-term survival on high impact palliative intent operations. Am J Surg 2020. https://doi.org/10.1016/j.amjsurg.2020.08.034.
38. Shimomura M, Toyota K, Karakuchi N, et al. Prognostic nutritional index predicts treatment outcomes following palliative surgery for colorectal adenocarcinoma. J Anus Rectum Colon 2017;1(4):118–24.
39. Roses RE, Tzeng C-WD, Ross MI, et al. The palliative index: predicting outcomes of emergent surgery in patients with cancer. J Palliat Med 2014;17(1):37–42.
40. Tseng WH, Yang X, Wang H, et al. Nomogram to predict risk of 30-day morbidity and mortality for patients with disseminated malignancy undergoing surgical intervention. Ann Surg 2011;254(2):333–8.
41. Vidri RJ, Blakely AM, Kulkarni SS, et al. American College of Surgeons National Surgical Quality Improvement Program as a quality-measurement tool for advanced cancer patients. Ann Palliat Med 2015;4(4):200–6.
42. Rodriguez RA, Fahy BN, McClain M, et al. Estimation of risk in cancer patients undergoing palliative procedures by the American College of Surgeons Risk Calculator. J Palliat Med 2016;19(10):1039–42.

Considerations in the Management of Malignant Bowel Obstruction

Caitlin T. Yeo, BSc, MD[a], Shaila J. Merchant, MSc, MHSc, MD, FRCSC[b],*

KEYWORDS

- Malignant bowel obstruction • Cancer • Palliative management • Medical therapy
- Surgery • Gastrostomy tube • Stents • Ablation

KEY POINTS

- Malignant bowel obstruction (MBO) is encountered in advanced intra-abdominal and pelvic malignancies and requires a patient-centered multidisciplinary approach. Specialized teams with expertise in symptom assessment and management are recommended.
- The existing literature is based predominantly on retrospective case series reporting survival as the primary outcome. Prospective studies that evaluate symptom relief and quality of life are under way.
- Medical treatment, including nasogastric tube decompression, intravenous fluids, and medications, are the mainstay of management.
- Procedural (venting gastrostomy tubes and stents) and surgical (resection, bypass, and stoma creation) interventions may be offered to well-selected patients.

BACKGROUND

Malignant bowel obstruction (MBO) is a challenging problem that patients and clinicians encounter in advanced malignancies and may occur in up to 51% of patients with colorectal, ovarian, pancreatic, and gastric cancers.[1] MBO can cause symptoms of abdominal pain, nausea, and vomiting and often requires hospitalization and has an impact on patient quality of life (QOL).[2] It usually represents a terminal phase of the disease with median survival in the range of 1 month to 3 months.[3] In 2007, the International Conference on Malignant Bowel Obstruction and the Clinical Protocol Committee proposed the following specific criteria for MBO: (1) clinical evidence of bowel obstruction, (2) bowel obstruction beyond the ligament of Treitz, and (3)

Funding: None.
[a] Division of Surgical Oncology, University of Calgary, Tom Baker Cancer Centre, 1331 29 St NW, Calgary, Alberta T2N 4N2, Canada; [b] Division of General Surgery and Surgical Oncology, Queen's University, Burr 2, 76 Stuart Street, Kingston, Ontario K7L 2V7, Canada
* Division of General Surgery and Surgical Oncology, Queen's University, Burr 2, 76 Stuart Street, Kingston, Ontario K7L 2V7, Canada
E-mail address: shaila.merchant@kingstonhsc.ca
Twitter: @QueensGenSurg (S.J.M.)

Surg Oncol Clin N Am 30 (2021) 461–474
https://doi.org/10.1016/j.soc.2021.02.003
1055-3207/21/

surgonc.theclinics.com

intraabdominal primary cancer with incurable disease, or (4) nonintraabdominal primary cancer with clear intraperitoneal disease.[4] These criteria are utilized by the authors and, therefore, the management of esophageal and gastric outlet obstruction is not discussed. Although benign causes of obstruction (ie, adhesions, hernia, and strictures) are important to consider, they are responsible for approximately 10% of obstructions in patients with a clinical suspicion of MBO[5] and are not related directly to malignancy; therefore, they are not discussed.

MBO comprises a wide variety of causative factors, including mechanical and functional causes and intraluminal and extraluminal sources, and may be related to primary or recurrent disease, nodal metastasis, or carcinomatosis.[6] Functional impairment can be due to tumor involvement of nerves in the mesentery or celiac plexus, chemotherapy and radiation side effects, opiate and anticholinergic medications, and electrolyte abnormalities due to dehydration, vomiting, and paraneoplastic syndromes.[6] Obstruction causes bowel wall distention, resulting in increased fluid secretion and release of inflammatory mediators and vasoactive intestinal polypeptide that further worsen bowel edema and symptoms of bloating, cramping, nausea, and vomiting.[7] Radiographic investigation is important in differentiating between functional and mechanical causes of MBO and determining the burden and level of disease. Plain films have poor sensitivity and specificity and are more useful for identifying constipation or assessing response to treatment.[8] Computed tomography has a sensitivity of 48% to 81%, depending on the degree of obstruction, and a specificity of up to 95% for identifying the cause[9] and plays a major role in guiding management decisions.[10]

The inability to tolerate oral intake has significant psychological and social implications for patients and their families. The goals of treatment must consider patient priorities and QOL. Often the most important goal for these patients is the ability to spend time with family at home[11]; however, a majority of studies reporting on MBO outcomes focus on overall survival and there is a lack of data that capture symptom relief and QOL.[12] Selecting the appropriate treatment of a patient with MBO is challenging and requires an individualized patient-centered multidisciplinary approach. Treatment may involve 1 or more medical, procedural, or surgical interventions. Realistic expectations regarding outcomes and potential risks of each treatment option require careful discussion. Providing the appropriate information and the manner in which it is conveyed is critical but may pose challenges for the health care provider. In a survey,[13] surgeons reported facing the ethical dilemma of "providing patients with honest information without destroying hope."

The objectives of this article are to (1) review the management of MBO summarizing medical, procedural, and surgical options using the currently available evidence and (2) highlight some new developments in the field.

MEDICAL MANAGEMENT

Medical therapies form the mainstay of management. This usually requires insertion of a nasogastric tube (NGT) for decompression and administration of a variety of agents, including intravenous fluids, analgesics, steroids, antisecretory, antimotility, and antiemetic agents, for which there are several existing reports.[1,6,14,15] There is limited evidence to support the use of water-soluble contrast agents to alleviate symptoms of MBO.[16] This section discusses studies that compare outcomes of medical management to surgical and procedural interventions.

A large population-based study compared surgical, procedural (gastrostomy tubes and stents), and medical management of MBO in patients with colorectal, gastric, ovarian, and pancreatic cancers in their final year of life.[17] A majority (65%) of patients received medical therapy alone compared with surgical and procedural management. Although those who received medical management had the shortest hospital length of stay (LOS), they also had the highest readmissions for obstruction. During the study period, the utilization of gastrostomy tubes and stents increased whereas the utilization of surgery decreased. Rates of medical management remained stable and high, suggesting that it is a mainstay in management. Bateni and colleagues[18] reported a greater utilization of medical (75%) compared with surgical (25%) strategies in patients with MBO. Medical management was associated with less hospital utilization, fewer in-hospital deaths, and more frequent discharges home; however, readmissions to hospital and rates of reobstruction were higher in patients managed medically. Lilley and colleagues[19] studied patients with MBO from ovarian or pancreatic cancer at the end of life and reported a high (69%) utilization of medical management; however, patients treated with surgery or gastrostomy tubes had lower risk of readmission for MBO. With respect to survival, some studies report increased survival associated with surgical compared with medical management[17,19] whereas other studies report no difference by management type.[18,20]

In summary, medical management is the mainstay of treatment of patients with MBO. Compared with surgical and procedural interventions, those managed medically have shorter hospital LOSs but also are more likely to be readmitted for resurgence in symptoms. Some patients may be good candidates for procedural and surgical interventions.

PROCEDURAL MANAGEMENT

In recent years, increased experience with procedural interventions, such as venting gastrostomy tube (VGT), endoscopic stent, and ablation, has added to the armamentarium of options to consider in the management of MBO.

Venting Gastrostomy Tubes

Experience with VGT for the management of MBO has increased over the years, with safe performance in increasingly complex patients. VGTs are inserted to relieve refractory nausea and vomiting, usually in the setting of multilevel obstruction and gut dysfunction, where surgery is not feasible, and generally in patients with limited life expectancy.[21] Successful insertion of VGT allows for removal of the NGT and can serve as a durable long-term management option. VGT can be placed surgically in the operating room, endoscopically, or under fluoroscopic guidance by interventional radiology, with recent reports favoring the endoscopic, fluoroscopic, and combined approaches.

Several case series[22–25] and a systematic review[26] report outcomes of VGT in patients with MBO. There is substantial variability in outcomes, which is expected, given the heterogeneity in the patient cohorts and definitions of complications. Richards and colleagues[24] reported a 9% major and 37% minor complication rate, whereas Shaw and colleagues[25] reported a 10% major and 4% minor complication rate. Overall, insertion of a VGT was found to significantly reduce the symptoms of nausea and vomiting.[22,23]

Patients with malignant ascites may have an increased likelihood of complications or unsuccessful VGT insertion[22,23]; however, successful placement was performed in 77% of patients in 1 study.[25] Insertion of a temporary or indwelling intraperitoneal catheter for ascites management may help to facilitate greater success of VGT insertion.[23,25] In a recent systematic review, which included 25 studies and 1194 patients, Thampy and colleagues[26] summarized a variety of outcomes related to VGT insertion, including successful insertion at first attempt in 91%, major complication in 2%, and minor complication in 20%. Furthermore, median survival ranged from 17 days to 74 days, and mean survival ranged from 35 days to 147 days, consistent with existing literature demonstrating poor survival in these patients.

In summary, insertion of a VGT is helpful in alleviating nausea and vomiting and can be performed safely. In patients with ascites, there is an increased likelihood of complications and unsuccessful insertion; however, ascites is not considered an absolute contraindication to insertion.

Endoscopic Stents

Experience with endoscopically placed stents is growing. Stents often are used as a bridge to curative intent surgery, primarily for patients with colorectal obstruction.[27] In patients who are not candidates for a curative intent approach, stents are used to alleviate symptoms of MBO related to a single point of obstruction. Patients with multilevel obstruction generally are not candidates for stent placement.

Some general considerations of stent placement include the availability of local expertise, site and length of the obstruction, use of covered versus uncovered stents, risk of complications, surgical options, patient prognosis, and the need for systemic therapy.[27,28] The European Society of Gastrointestinal Endoscopy[28] and America Society for Gastrointestinal Endoscopy[27] suggest that stent placement is effective for palliation of colonic MBO. Placement of stents for this indication is associated with high rates of clinical success, shorter hospitalization, decreased intensive care unit admission, and shorter time to initiation of chemotherapy, but a higher risk of long-term complications, such as perforation, migration, and reobstruction compared with surgery, demonstrated in 2 separate meta-analyses.[29,30] A randomized clinical trial comparing endoscopic stent to surgery for metastatic left-sided colorectal cancer closed early because of a greater than expected rate of perforation in the stent group.[31]

The majority of experience with endoscopic stents comes from stenting intraluminal lesions due to colorectal cancer rather than narrowing or invasion secondary to extraluminal pathology. Single-institution studies have examined the use of stents in extraluminal narrowing secondary to genitourinary, gynecologic, pancreatic, and gastric cancers.[32–34] In these small studies, technical success was reported to be 87% to 90% in 2 of the studies[33,34] but was low (20%) in another study that compared outcomes in patients receiving stents for colonic versus extracolonic malignancy.[32] In that study, patients with extracolonic malignancy were more likely to require surgical diversion for persistent obstructive symptoms despite stent insertion.[32] In a large multicenter study, extrinsic compression from tumor also was associated with a higher likelihood of technical and clinical failure.[35] Overall, there are few data to support the use of stents in extracolonic malignancies.

Another important consideration is the increased risk of stent perforation in patients receiving antiangiogenic agents as part of systemic therapy. In a meta-analysis, the use of bevacizumab was associated with a 12.5% risk of perforation compared with 7% in patients receiving chemotherapy without bevacizumab.[36] A 20-fold increase in stent perforation with bevacizumab also was reported by a multicenter Italian study.[35] Therefore, decision making surrounding stent placement also should include consideration of systemic therapies that a patient may be eligible for.

Finally, the risk of stent complication is higher in patients who live longer with the stent[29,30]; therefore, patients with a longer life expectancy may be considered for surgery. Manes and colleagues[35] reported, however, that 82% of stents maintained patency at 6 months, and 65% still were functioning 1 year after placement. Taken together, the selection of patients who are suitable for stent placement requires a careful discussion of risks and benefits and the consideration of potential systemic therapies and patient prognosis.

Endoscopic Ablative Therapies

The utilization of endoscopic ablative therapies to palliate symptoms (ie, obstruction, pain, and bleeding) from carcinomas of the gastrointestinal tract is reported in patients who are deemed unfit for surgery, but the literature is outdated. Commonly described modalities for palliation of lower gastrointestinal tract cancers are Nd:YAG[37–42] and diode,[43] which are forms of laser ablation and typically require multiple treatment sessions. Reported complications include perforation, stricture, and hemorrhage.[39]

Farouk and colleagues[37] reported outcomes in a small series of patients receiving Nd:YAG in the palliation of advanced rectal cancer. This was successful as the sole form of treatment in 78% of patients, with 76% avoiding an ostomy. Eckhauser and Mansour[40] reported successful palliation of obstructive symptoms with decreased hospital LOS and overall cost in patients treated with the Nd:YAG laser compared with operative diversion in patients eligible for a staged resection of their colorectal malignancy. In patients who were deemed to have unresectable disease, the same investigators reported successful palliation of obstructive and bleeding symptoms. Van Cutsem and colleagues[42] reported that although initial palliation was achieved in 88% of patients, it could be maintained only in 51% and 41% of patients at 6 months and 12 months, respectively. Use of diode laser demonstrates similar outcomes for initial palliation, with the advantages of smaller size, portability, and lower cost over Nd:YAG laser.[43]

In summary, the experience with endoscopic ablative therapies for palliation of lower gastrointestinal tract malignancies is outdated, and utilization is highly dependent on availability of the necessary equipment and expertise. There is a need for updated literature.

SURGICAL MANAGEMENT
Outcomes of Surgery

Decisions pertaining to the surgical management of MBO are challenging, and current recommendations are based mainly on retrospective cohort or case series data. In 2016, an updated Cochrane review was performed regarding surgery for MBO in patients with advanced gastrointestinal and gynecologic cancers.[12] Since the initial review performed in 2000,[44] none of the new studies provided additional information to change the original conclusions. The investigators reported high risk of bias in the studies that were included, most of which were retrospective case series. There was a lack of standardized outcome measures, no data available on QOL, and marked variation in clinical management. They concluded that the role of surgery for MBO requires careful evaluation using validated outcome measures and that a greater standardization in management should be considered.

Olson and colleagues[45] performed a systematic review of patients undergoing surgery for MBO from peritoneal carcinomatosis. The data were heterogeneous and the results were highly variable. They found that surgery led to symptom improvement in 32% to 100%, resumption of diet in 45% to 75%, and facilitated discharge home in 34% to 87%. Mortality ranged from 6% to 32% and major morbidity from 7% to 44%. Persistent and recurrent obstruction and readmissions due to MBO were up to 47%, with all-cause readmission rates as high as 74%. Furthermore, median survival was limited, particularly in those with poor prognostic features (ie, ascites, palpable mass, and continued obstruction postoperatively) who survived only

26 days to 36 days. A study by Bateni and colleagues[18] also reported that patients treated with surgery had higher rates of complications (44% vs 21%), in-hospital deaths (10% vs 4%), and lower rates of discharge home (76% vs 90%) compared with patients receiving medical management. Furthermore, patients who experience a major postoperative complication are less likely to experience improvement in symptoms.[46] The survival benefit associated with surgical management reported by some[17,19] is likely a result of selection bias, whereby patients with better performance status and favorable disease are selected to undergo surgery and ultimately have better outcomes. These studies highlight that although surgery may lead to symptom improvement and survival benefit in some, it is associated with substantial morbidity and mortality and lower rates of discharge home.

Patient Selection Strategies

Patients with MBO are at high risk of complications from surgery due to the increasing burden of cancer, cancer-related catabolism, and malnutrition caused by the insidious progression of their MBO.[47] Despite these risks, there still may be a role for surgical management in appropriately selected patients because some tolerate palliative surgery and chemotherapy with survival beyond 1 year.[48]

Multiple studies have reported on factors that are associated with poor surgical outcomes. Wright and colleagues[3] reported that patients with an Eastern Cooperative Oncology Group (ECOG) score of 0 or 1 had a mean survival of 7.5 months compared with 1 months to 2 months in patients with an ECOG score of 2 or greater, regardless of medical and/or surgical intervention. Surgery does not benefit patients with poor clinical status, multilevel obstruction, ascites, carcinomatosis, palpable masses, or very advanced disease. Rather, these patients are better palliated with medical management or VGT.[49] Studies suggest that any ascites is a predictor of poor outcome, high recurrence rates, and increased morbidity and mortality.[50,51] One retrospective study found that low serum albumin, metachronous presentation of cancer and obstruction, ECOG score greater than 1, and low hematocrit on admission were predictive of 90-day mortality in patients with stage 4 cancer undergoing surgery for MBO.[52]

Anticipating who is most likely to benefit from surgical intervention is critical. Diagnostic laparoscopy may allow for a more accurate assessment of disease burden to identify those that may benefit from surgery.[53] Sugarbaker[54] recommended surgical intervention in patients with good performance status, localized disease, and low histologic grade. Krebs and Goplerud[55] developed a prognostic index and reported that patients less than 45 years old with minimal nutritional deficiency, no palpable intraabdominal masses, little to no ascites, no progression while on chemotherapy, and no prior radiation therapy had improved outcomes after surgery. Other factors that influence a surgeon's choice to offer surgical intervention include younger patient age, low-grade or indolent tumors, good preoperative functional status, and potential for symptom control.[13] These studies are limited by their retrospective nature and lack of explicit patient selection strategies. Prospective studies are needed to better define prognostic factors and outcomes for patients undergoing surgical intervention for MBO.

Surgical Options

The surgical options for MBO include resection, bypass, stoma creation, and VGTs. Surgical resection of the obstruction is ideal if there is localized disease in an area that can be removed; however, in a population-based study by Merchant and colleagues,[17] only 10% of surgically managed MBO patients underwent resection. Bypass surgery allows for successful palliation[56] and is selected when resection is not possible due to dense adhesions or significant lengths of affected bowel. This often is encountered in patients who have had previous radiotherapy.[57] If resection or bypass is possible and an anastomosis is created, it is important to consider the nutritional status of the patient and its implications on healing because malnutrition is an independent risk factor for anastomotic leak.[58] Creation of a stoma is considered when the obstruction involves the distal small bowel or colon and when anastomotic healing is a concern. Proximal obstructions are not amenable to stomas due to problems of high output, dehydration and electrolyte imbalance.[59] Finally, if the intraoperative findings are worse than expected and resection, bypass, or stoma creation is not possible, placement of a VGT may allow for decompression and symptom management.[26] Laparoscopic approaches to MBO may be a less-invasive option with potential for lower morbidity,[56] but this is likely approach inappropriate for patients with extremely distended bowel, significant burden of disease, or dense adhesions from prior surgery, because there is an increased risk of iatrogenic injury.[60] Merchant and colleagues[17] reported that only 5% of patients had laparoscopic surgery for MBO.

In summary, surgical decision making in MBO requires a tailored multidisciplinary approach that should consider expected outcomes of surgery, appropriate patient selection, and the ideal intraoperative approach, with alternative plans for palliation if the extent of disease is greater than anticipated. Specific considerations include location and extent of disease, disease cadence, overall prognosis, patient nutritional status and comorbidities, availability of life-extending systemic therapy, previous administration of radiotherapy, and patient preferences and goals of care. Although surgical intervention may provide symptom relief in well-selected patients, it is associated with substantial morbidity and mortality, and at the current time there is a lack of high-level evidence for or against surgery for MBO.[12]

NEW DEVELOPMENTS AND FUTURE DIRECTIONS
Multidisciplinary Management and Opportunities for Palliative Care

With high symptom burden, frequent hospitalizations, limited life span, and complexities surrounding patient goals of care and QOL, patients with MBO may be managed best by providers with appropriate expertise. This is well demonstrated in a study by Lee and colleagues,[61] which describes the experience of a Canadian hospital that developed a dedicated multidisciplinary team that reviews and manages all MBO cases in gynecologic cancer patients. After program implementation, women with MBO spent less time in hospital and had fewer intensive care unit admissions. They also were less likely to undergo palliative surgery but more likely to undergo chemotherapy. MBO resolution rates were similar among the groups. The investigators suggested that a specialized program for this high-needs population improved the care and outcomes of these patients. A study by Miner and colleagues[62] demonstrated that open dialogue between the surgeon, patient, and family in key decision making pertaining to palliative surgery led to improved patient outcomes, including high rates of symptom resolution and fewer postoperative complications compared with the published literature at that time. These studies demonstrate the clear benefits of appropriate expertise in the management of patients with MBO.

Consideration of referral to a palliative care service is also reasonable, given the high symptom burden and proximity to death. Prior studies have shown very low rates of referral to palliative care.[19] A recent randomized clinical trial demonstrated that close symptom monitoring of patients with cancer, in whom worsening symptoms triggered a specific intervention resulted in improved median survival compared with those who received usual care.[63] Gabriel and colleagues[64] reported that patients with MBO who were managed by a palliative care service had greater improvement in symptoms,

Table 1
General considerations for medical, procedural and surgical interventions for malignant bowel obstruction

Intervention	General Considerations
Medical	1. Typically the mainstay of management[17,18] 2. Patient not suitable for procedure or surgery 3. Patient has limited life span 4. Hospital LOS is short but readmissions for obstruction are high[17,18]
Procedural	1. Patient has obstruction amenable to procedural intervention 2. Appropriate expertise available 3. Patient understands risks, benefits, and limitations of the procedure 4. Lower risk of readmission for obstruction compared with medical management[19]
Surgical	1. Patient has obstruction amenable to surgical intervention 2. Appropriate expertise available 3. Reasonable expectation that the patient will tolerate surgical intervention 4. Patient understands risks, benefits, and limitations of the surgery 5. Increased survival compared with medical management[17,19,62] 6. Higher rates of complications, in-hospital deaths, and lower rates of discharge home compared with medical management[18]

higher rates of documentation of do-not-resuscitate wishes, and higher rates of discharge to hospice compared with those who did not have involvement of a palliative care service. These studies suggest benefit to close symptom monitoring and management, best done by multidisciplinary teams with appropriate expertise.

Measuring the Success of Interventions and Upcoming Studies

There is a need to consider outcomes beyond survival and complications, which traditionally are reported in the MBO literature.[65,66] Survival is less relevant because these patients typically have a short life expectancy. Complications are important to report but provide only a glimpse of the whole picture. QOL-centered and patient-reported outcomes, including ability to return home or to a hospice, days out of hospital,

Table 2
Patient selection and outcomes of procedural interventions for malignant bowel obstruction

Procedural Intervention	Patient Selection	Outcomes
Venting gastrostomy tube	Multilevel obstruction Gut dysfunction Patients with ascites may be considered[25]	Successful insertion at first attempt = 91%[26] Major complication = 2%[26] Minor complication = 20%[26]
Endoscopic stents	Single site of obstruction Intraluminal obstruction Higher risk of perforation in patients receiving bevacizumab[35,36]	Technical success at first attempt = 92%[35] Successful colonic decompression = 90%[35] 6-mo stent patency = 82%[35] 1-y stent patency = 65%[35] Stent migration = 9%[30] Stent perforation = 10%[30] Stent occlusion = 18%[30]
Endoscopic ablative therapies	Patients with bleeding, obstruction, tenesmus	Avoidance of ostomy = 76%[37]

good days, days without NGT, resumption of oral intake, relief of nausea and vomiting, QOL scores, need for total parenteral nutrition, and readmission for obstruction, must be considered. Determining the success of treatment requires careful consideration of some or all of these outcomes, and future research endeavors must consider these.

Review of several clinical trials currently recruiting patients with MBO reveals that more relevant outcomes are indeed being considered. For example, the Southwest Oncology Group S136 prospective randomized trial (NCT02270450) is comparing surgical to nonsurgical management and will examine outcomes, such as days outside hospital, ability to eat, days with NGT, intravenous hydration, solid food, and survival. A single-arm prospective study from Roswell Park Cancer Institute (NCT04027348) is examining the efficacy of triple therapy with dexamethasone, octreotide, and metoclopramide in clearing obstruction. The MAMBO trial (NCT03260647) is a prospective study that is aiming to streamline the management of MBO in patients with advanced gynecologic cancer through development of a multidisciplinary team and algorithm for outpatient management. These trials are anticipated to provide high-level evidence to inform clinical decision making.

Table 3
Prognostic factors, patient selection, and outcomes for surgical interventions for malignant bowel obstruction

Prognostic Factors/ Surgical Intervention	Patient Selection	Outcomes
Prognostic factors associated with benefit from surgery	Age <45 y, minimal nutritional deficiency, no palpable intraabdominal masses, little to no ascites, no progression while on chemotherapy, low-grade localized disease, good performance status, reasonable life expectancy[13,54,55]	Mortality = 6%–32%[45] Serious complications = 7%–44%[45] Recurrent obstruction = 0–63%[12] Palliation of obstructive symptoms = 32%–100%[45] Increased survival compared with medical management[17,19,62] Fewer readmissions for obstruction compared with medical management = 25% vs 33%[19]
Resection	Localized disease Good nutritional status	Restores bowel continuity Avoids ostomy Risk of anastomotic leak
Bypass	Dense adhesions or significant lengths of affected bowel Irradiated bowel[57]	Restores bowel continuity without resection Avoids ostomy Risk of anastomotic leak
Ostomy	Distal small bowel or colorectal obstruction Emergent/impending perforation Concerning nutritional status[58]	Avoids risk of anastomotic leak Risk of high-output ostomy requiring hospital admission = 26%–37%[59] Short-term (retraction, necrosis, skin irritation, leakage) and long-term (prolapse, hernia, body perception) complications of ostomy

SUMMARY

A 1-size-fits-all approach is not suitable for patients suffering from MBO. A variety of management options are available, and the optimal approach must consider patient suitability for procedural or surgical interventions, performance status, prognosis, preferences, goals of care, QOL, and the availability of local expertise. General considerations, patient selection, and outcomes of medical, procedural, and surgical interventions are summarized in **Tables 1–3.**

Given that MBO is considered a preterminal event with poor survival, future research endeavors must move away from outcomes, such as survival, and consider more relevant, patient-centered outcomes. Results from the prospective trials, discussed previously, are expected to provide higher-level evidence than exist currently. There is emerging evidence that multidisciplinary teams with expertise in symptom evaluation and management are best suited to manage these patients and consideration should be given to assembling such teams at local institutions.

CLINICS CARE POINTS

- Medical interventions are the foundation of management in MBO.
- Some patients may have disease that is amenable to procedural and/or surgical interventions.
- If procedural and/or surgical interventions are deemed reasonable, the appropriate expertise must be available, and the patient should have a clear understanding of the risks, benefits, and limitations of the proposed plan.
- Evidence suggests that the involvement of multidisciplinary teams with interest and expertise in MBO can improve patient outcomes.

DISCLOSURE

The authors have nothing to disclose.

REFERENCES

1. Tuca A, Guell E, Martinez-Losada E, et al. Malignant bowel obstruction in advanced cancer patients: epidemiology, management, and factors influencing spontaneous resolution. Cancer Manag Res 2012;4:159–69.
2. Gwilliam B, Bailey C. The nature of terminal malignant bowel obstruction and its impact on patients with advanced cancer. Int J Palliat Nurs 2001;7(10):474–81.
3. Wright FC, Chakraborty A, Helyer L, et al. Predictors of survival in patients with non-curative stage IV cancer and malignant bowel obstruction. J Surg Oncol 2010;101(5):425–9.
4. Anthony T, Baron T, Mercadante S, et al. Report of the clinical protocol committee: development of randomized trials for malignant bowel obstruction. J Pain Symptom Manag 2007;34(1 Suppl):S49–59.
5. Legendre H, Vanhuyse F, Caroli-Bosc FX, et al. Survival and quality of life after palliative surgery for neoplastic gastrointestinal obstruction. Eur J Surg Oncol 2001;27(4):364–7.
6. Ripamonti CI, Easson AM, Gerdes H. Management of malignant bowel obstruction. Eur J Cancer 2008;44(8):1105–15.
7. Nellgard P, Bojo L, Cassuto J. Importance of vasoactive intestinal peptide and somatostatin for fluid losses in small-bowel obstruction. Scand J Gastroenterol 1995;30(5):464–9.

8. Maglinte D, Kelvin F, Sandrasegaran K, et al. Radiology of small bowel obstruction: contemporary approach and controversies. Abdom Imaging 2005;30(2): 160–78.
9. Maglinte DD, Heitkamp DE, Howard TJ, et al. Current concepts in imaging of small bowel obstruction. Radiologic Clin 2003;41(2):263–83.
10. Silva AC, Pimenta M, Guimaraes LS. Small bowel obstruction: what to look for. Radiographics 2009;29(2):423–39.
11. Higginson IJ, Sen-Gupta G. Place of care in advanced cancer: a qualitative systematic literature review of patient preferences. J Palliat Med 2000;3(3):287–300.
12. Cousins SE, Tempest E, Feuer DJ. Surgery for the resolution of symptoms in malignant bowel obstruction in advanced gynaecological and gastrointestinal cancer. Cochrane Database Syst Rev 2016;(1):CD002764.
13. McCahill LE, Krouse RS, Chu DZ, et al. Decision making in palliative surgery. J Am Coll Surg 2002;195(3):411–22.
14. Franke AJ, Iqbal A, Starr JS, et al. Management of malignant bowel obstruction associated with GI cancers. J Oncol Pract 2017;13(7):426–34.
15. Laval G, Marcelin-Benazech B, Guirimand F, et al. Recommendations for bowel obstruction with peritoneal carcinomatosis. J Pain Symptom Manag 2014;48(1): 75–91.
16. Syrmis W, Richard R, Jenkins-Marsh S, et al. Oral water soluble contrast for malignant bowel obstruction. Cochrane Database Syst Rev 2018;(3):CD012014.
17. Merchant SJ, Brogly SB, Booth CM, et al. Management of cancer-associated intestinal obstruction in the final year of life. J Palliat Care 2020;35(2):84–92.
18. Bateni SB, Gingrich AA, Stewart SL, et al. Hospital utilization and disposition among patients with malignant bowel obstruction: a population-based comparison of surgical to medical management. BMC Cancer 2018;18(1):1166.
19. Lilley EJ, Scott JW, Goldberg JE, et al. Survival, healthcare utilization, and end-of-life care among older adults with malignancy-associated bowel obstruction: comparative study of surgery, venting gastrostomy, or medical management. Ann Surg 2018;267(4):692–9.
20. Winner M, Mooney SJ, Hershman DL, et al. Management and outcomes of bowel obstruction in patients with stage IV colon cancer: a population-based cohort study. Dis Colon rectum 2013;56(7):834–43.
21. National Comprehensive Cancer Network (NCCN). Palliative Care Version 1 2020. Available at: https://www.nccn.org/professionals/physician_gls/default.aspx#supportive. Accessed July 2, 2020.
22. Dittrich A, Schubert B, Kramer M, et al. Benefits and risks of a percutaneous endoscopic gastrostomy (PEG) for decompression in patients with malignant gastrointestinal obstruction. Support Care Cancer 2017;25(9):2849–56.
23. Issaka RB, Shapiro DM, Parikh ND, et al. Palliative venting percutaneous endoscopic gastrostomy tube is safe and effective in patients with malignant obstruction. Surg Endosc 2014;28(5):1668–73.
24. Richards DM, Tanikella R, Arora G, et al. Percutaneous endoscopic gastrostomy in cancer patients: predictors of 30-day complications, 30-day mortality, and overall mortality. Dig Dis Sci 2013;58(3):768–76.
25. Shaw C, Bassett RL, Fox PS, et al. Palliative venting gastrostomy in patients with malignant bowel obstruction and ascites. Ann Surg Oncol 2013;20(2):497–505.
26. Thampy S, Najran P, Mullan D, et al. Safety and efficacy of venting gastrostomy in malignant bowel obstruction: a systematic review. J Palliat Care 2020;35(2): 93–102.

27. American Society of Gastrointestinal Endoscopy Standards of Practice Committee, Harrison ME, Anderson MA, Appalaneni V, et al. The role of endoscopy in the management of patients with known and suspected colonic obstruction and pseudo-obstruction. Gastrointest Endosc 2010;71(4):669–79.

28. van Hooft JE, van Halsema EE, Vanbiervliet G, et al. Self-expandable metal stents for obstructing colonic and extracolonic cancer: European Society of Gastrointestinal Endoscopy (ESGE) Clinical Guideline. Gastrointest Endosc 2014;80(5): 747–61.e1-75.

29. Liang TW, Sun Y, Wei YC, et al. Palliative treatment of malignant colorectal obstruction caused by advanced malignancy: a self-expanding metallic stent or surgery? A system review and meta-analysis. Surg Today 2014;44(1):22–33.

30. Zhao XD, Cai BB, Cao RS, et al. Palliative treatment for incurable malignant colorectal obstructions: a meta-analysis. World J Gastroenterol 2013;19(33):5565–74.

31. van Hooft JE, Fockens P, Marinelli AW, et al. Early closure of a multicenter randomized clinical trial of endoscopic stenting versus surgery for stage IV left-sided colorectal cancer. Endoscopy 2008;40(3):184–91.

32. Keswani RN, Azar RR, Edmundowicz SA, et al. Stenting for malignant colonic obstruction: a comparison of efficacy and complications in colonic versus extracolonic malignancy. Gastrointest Endosc 2009;69(3 Pt 2):675–80.

33. Kim JH, Ku YS, Jeon TJ, et al. The efficacy of self-expanding metal stents for malignant colorectal obstruction by noncolonic malignancy with peritoneal carcinomatosis. Dis Colon rectum 2013;56(11):1228–32.

34. Shin SJ, Kim TI, Kim BC, et al. Clinical application of self-expandable metallic stent for treatment of colorectal obstruction caused by extrinsic invasive tumors. Dis Colon rectum 2008;51(5):578–83.

35. Manes G, de Bellis M, Fuccio L, et al. Endoscopic palliation in patients with incurable malignant colorectal obstruction by means of self-expanding metal stent: analysis of results and predictors of outcomes in a large multicenter series. Arch Surg 2011;146(10):1157–62.

36. van Halsema EE, van Hooft JE, Small AJ, et al. Perforation in colorectal stenting: a meta-analysis and a search for risk factors. Gastrointest Endosc 2014;79(6): 970–82.e7 [quiz: 83.e2, e5].

37. Farouk R, Ratnaval CD, Monson JR, et al. Staged delivery of Nd:YAG laser therapy for palliation of advanced rectal carcinoma. Dis Colon rectum 1997;40(2): 156–60.

38. Eckhauser ML. Laser therapy of gastrointestinal tumors. World J Surg 1992;16(6): 1054–9.

39. Eckhauser ML. Laser therapy of colorectal carcinoma. Surg Clin North Am 1992; 72(3):597–607.

40. Eckhauser ML, Mansour EG. Endoscopic laser therapy for obstructing and/or bleeding colorectal carcinoma. Am Surg 1992;58(6):358–63.

41. Schwesinger WH, Chumley DL. Laser palliation for gastrointestinal malignancy. Am Surg 1988;54(2):100–4.

42. Van Cutsem E, Boonen A, Geboes K, et al. Risk factors which determine the long term outcome of Neodymium-YAG laser palliation of colorectal carcinoma. Int J Colorectal Dis 1989;4(1):9–11.

43. Courtney ED, Raja A, Leicester RJ. Eight years experience of high-powered endoscopic diode laser therapy for palliation of colorectal carcinoma. Dis Colon rectum 2005;48(4):845–50.

44. Feuer DJ, Broadley KE, Shepherd JH, et al. Surgery for the resolution of symptoms in malignant bowel obstruction in advanced gynaecological and gastrointestinal cancer. Cochrane Database Syst Rev 2000;(4):CD002764.
45. Olson TJP, Pinkerton C, Brasel KJ, et al. Palliative surgery for malignant bowel obstruction from carcinomatosis: a systematic review. JAMA Surg 2014;149(4): 383–92.
46. Miner TJ, Brennan MF, Jaques DP. A prospective, symptom related, outcomes analysis of 1022 palliative procedures for advanced cancer. Ann Surg 2004; 240(4):719.
47. Nicolini A, Ferrari P, Masoni MC, et al. Malnutrition, anorexia and cachexia in cancer patients: a mini-review on pathogenesis and treatment. Biomed Pharmacother 2013;67(8):807–17.
48. Helyer LK, Law CH, Butler M, et al. Surgery as a bridge to palliative chemotherapy in patients with malignant bowel obstruction from colorectal cancer. Ann Surg Oncol 2007;14(4):1264–71.
49. Ripamonti C. Management of bowel obstruction in advanced cancer. Curr Opin Oncol 1994;6(4):351–7.
50. Blair SL, Chu DZ, Schwarz RE. Outcome of palliative operations for malignant bowel obstruction in patients with peritoneal carcinomatosis from nongynecological cancer. Ann Surg Oncol 2001;8(8):632–7.
51. Krouse RS, McCahill LE, Easson AM, et al. When the sun can set on an unoperated bowel obstruction: management of malignant bowel obstruction. J Am Coll Surg 2002;195(1):117–28.
52. Francescutti V, Miller A, Satchidanand Y, et al. Management of bowel obstruction in patients with stage IV cancer: predictors of outcome after surgery. Ann Surg Oncol 2013;20(3):707–14.
53. DeBernardo R. Surgical management of malignant bowel obstruction: strategies toward palliation of patients with advanced cancer. Curr Oncol Rep 2009;11(4): 287–92.
54. Sugarbaker P. Peritoneal surface oncology: review of a personal experience with colorectal and appendiceal malignancy. Tech Coloproctol 2005;9(2):95–103.
55. Krebs H-B, Goplerud DR. Surgical management of bowel obstruction in advanced ovarian carcinoma. Obstet Gynecol 1983;61(3):327–30.
56. Krouse RS. Surgical palliation of bowel obstruction. Gastroenterol Clin North Am 2006;35(1):143–51.
57. Lillemoe KD, Brigham RA, Harmon JW, et al. Surgical management of small-bowel radiation enteritis. Arch Surg 1983;118(8):905–7.
58. Lee SY, Jung MR, Kim CH, et al. Nutritional risk screening score is an independent predictive factor of anastomotic leakage after rectal cancer surgery. Eur J Clin Nutr 2018;72(4):489–95.
59. Justiniano CF, Temple LK, Swanger AA, et al. Readmissions with dehydration after ileostomy creation: rethinking risk factors. Dis Colon rectum 2018;61(11):1297.
60. Behman R, Nathens AB, Byrne JP, et al. Laparoscopic surgery for adhesive small bowel obstruction is associated with a higher risk of bowel injury: a population-based analysis of 8584 patients. Ann Surg 2017;266(3):489–98.
61. Lee YC, Jivraj N, Wang L, et al. Optimizing the care of malignant bowel obstruction in patients with advanced gynecologic cancer. J Oncol Pract 2019;15(12): e1066–75.
62. Miner TJ, Cohen J, Charpentier K, et al. The palliative triangle: improved patient selection and outcomes associated with palliative operations. Arch Surg 2011; 146(5):517–22.

63. Basch E, Deal AM, Dueck AC, et al. Overall survival results of a trial assessing patient-reported outcomes for symptom monitoring during routine cancer treatment. JAMA 2017;318(2):197–8.
64. Gabriel E, Kukar M, Groman A, et al. A formal palliative care service improves the quality of care in patients with stage IV cancer and bowel obstruction. Am J Hosp Palliat Care 2017;34(1):20–5.
65. Badgwell B, Krouse R, Klimberg SV, et al. Outcome measures other than morbidity and mortality for patients with incurable cancer and gastrointestinal obstruction. J Palliat Med 2014;17(1):18–26.
66. Krouse RS. The international conference on malignant bowel obstruction: a meeting of the minds to advance palliative care research. J Pain Symptom Manag 2007;34(1 Suppl):S1–6.

A Palliative Approach to Management of Peritoneal Carcinomatosis and Malignant Ascites

Josh Bleicher, MD MS*, Laura A. Lambert, MD

KEYWORDS

- Peritoneal carcinomatosis • Palliative care • Malignant bowel obstruction
- Malignant ascites • Cancer • Malignancy • Oncology

KEY POINTS

- Palliative care teams should be involved early in a multidisciplinary approach to care for patients with peritoneal carcinomatosis.
- A variety of medical, interventional, and surgical interventions are available for palliative treatment of complications of peritoneal carcinomatosis and should be considered based on individual patient goals, preferences, and disease characteristics.
- Surgical interventions in patients with peritoneal carcinomatosis can be accompanied by a higher risk, but can often offer excellent palliative treatment in appropriately selected patients.

INTRODUCTION

Peritoneal carcinomatosis (PC), the intraperitoneal spread of cancer, can be caused by both primary malignancy of the peritoneal lining of the abdomen and the metastatic spread of a cancer to the peritoneum. Drs Miller and Wynn first described PC in 1908 in a 32-year-old man who presented with 6 weeks of increasing abdominal girth.[1] At this time, and for many decades after, this represented an incurable and terminal clinical situation. Modern therapies for PC, including cytoreductive surgery and intraperitoneal chemotherapy, have offered patients prolonged survival and in some cases hope for a cure. Despite these significant advances, PC remains an extremely challenging disease for patients and providers, and is associated with low survival rates and high morbidity.

Division of General Surgery, Huntsman Cancer Institute, University of Utah, 1950 Circle of Hope, Suite 6405, Salt Lake City, UT 84112, USA
* Corresponding author. 30 N 1900 E, Salt Lake City, UT 84132.
E-mail address: Josh.bleicher@hsc.utah.edu

Surg Oncol Clin N Am 30 (2021) 475–490
https://doi.org/10.1016/j.soc.2021.02.004
1055-3207/21/© 2021 Elsevier Inc. All rights reserved.

surgonc.theclinics.com

After a diagnosis of PC, many patients experience significant symptoms impacting their quality of life, including pain, nausea, anorexia, cachexia, and fatigue. In addition, patients with PC often have major complications, such as functional and mechanical bowel obstructions, biliary and ureteral obstructions, enteric fistulae, and malignant ascites. Managing the complications and complexities of patients with PC requires not only specialized medical knowledge, but also attention to patient's unique psychological, social, and existential situations. For this reason, early referral to a comprehensive palliative care team is essential.

In this article, we present an updated review of the therapeutic options for patients with PC and malignant ascites from a palliative care perspective.

EARLY INVOLVEMENT OF PALLIATIVE CARE

The American Society of Clinical Oncology and the National Comprehensive Cancer Network guidelines recommend palliative care for all patients with advanced cancer, beginning at the time of diagnosis.[2,3] The Chicago Consensus on Peritoneal Surface Malignancies also suggests early involvement of palliative care.[4,5] Early involvement of a palliative care team has multiple benefits. First, early involvement allows patients to see palliative care as a normal part of their medical care, not as their doctors "giving up" as hope for a cure diminishes. Second, early palliative care involvement allows for patients to be introduced gradually to the worst case scenario, addressing their own mortality, while still allowing for hope. A visual way of understanding this concept is the bow tie model, introduced by Hawley[6] (**Fig. 1**).

Palliative care also allows for assistance with advance care planning (ACP). ACP includes not only ensuring that patients have updated advance directives and identified surrogate decision makers, but also engaging with the patient and their family in ongoing conversations about curative and palliative treatment options, the overall goals of care, and preferences on specific therapies such as life support or resuscitation.[7] Patients who participate in ACP are more likely to receive care aligned with their preferences at the end of life and family members are more likely to report improvements in end-of-life care and improved communication with providers.[8–10] The prognosis, quality of life, and available therapeutic options for patients with advanced

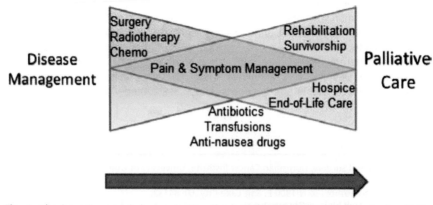

Fig. 1. The bow-tie model demonstrating the benefits of early involvement of palliative care. (*From* Hawley PH. The bow tie model of 21st century palliative care. *J Pain Symptom Manage.* 2014;47(1):2-5. https://doi.org/10.1016/j.jpainsymman.2013.10.009 with permission from Elsevier.)

cancer can change frequently, and early ACP can help to guide patients and their families as their experience living with advanced cancer evolves.

PALLIATING SYMPTOMS: PAIN, NAUSEA, VOMITING, CACHEXIA, FATIGUE, AND ANHEDONIA

Approximately 20% to 60% of patients with PC experience significant abdominal pain.[11,12] Some patients, particularly women with PC related to ovarian cancer, can also experience significant back pain.[13] The pain can be related to the disease itself and/or the therapeutic interventions used. The World Health Organization's analgesic ladder is an effective method for controlling pain in the majority of patients.[14] This process involves increasing the intensity of pain management in a step-wise fashion if pain is uncontrolled with the lowest level of treatment. The World Health Organization's ladder recommends the use of nonopioid analgesics (ie, acetaminophen, aspirin, and ibuprofen) for step 1, mild cancer pain. Lower potency opioids such as oxycodone, hydrocodone, or codeine are recommended for step 2, moderate pain. Highly potent opioids such as morphine, fentanyl, hydromorphone, and methadone are recommended for step 3, severe cancer pain. Other investigators have proposed the addition of a fourth rung to the ladder for invasive or minimally invasive pain therapies (ie, epidural analgesia, nerve ablation, nerve blocks, intrathecal anesthesia, etc) for pain refractory to the previously mentioned therapies.[15] The use of multimodal therapy, including the therapies mentioned and nonpharmacologic therapies (ie, physical therapy, acupuncture, relaxation techniques, and psychological support), should all be used as appropriate for individual patients.[16] The management of pain in patients with PC is sometimes further complicated by the inability to use an oral route of medication administration, because the intestinal tract is often unable to contribute to absorption. Other routes of medication administration, such as transdermal, subcutaneous, sublingual, or intramuscular, should be considered. Patients with refractory or difficult-to-manage pain may benefit from a pain specialist or palliative care consultation.

Nausea and vomiting also commonly affect patients with PC, particularly patients with bowel dysmotility or obstruction. A number of medical interventions are available for management of these symptoms. Nausea should be treated aggressively with broad-spectrum antiemetics, used in combination if necessary, to relieve symptoms. These agents include neuroleptic medications such as haloperidol and chlorpromazine, serotonin receptor antagonists like ondansetron, and antisecretory agents such as butylscopolamine (**Table 1**).[17,18] Somatostatin analogues, such as octreotide or lanreotide, have also been shown to be effective at decreasing nausea and the frequency of vomiting episodes through a decrease in intestinal secretions and bowel motility.[19,20] Corticosteroids, either methylprednisolone or dexamethasone, can be used to alleviate nausea, and also potentially relieve the underlying obstruction.[21,22] Corticosteroids act by decreasing edema surrounding a tumor, leading to decreased intestinal stenosis. Finally, gastric antisecretory medications such as proton pump inhibitors (ie, omeprazole) and H_2-blockers (ie, ranitidine) are recommended in the setting of malignant bowel obstruction to decrease upper gastrointestinal symptoms.[17,23] The initial choice of antiemetic should be focused on the underlying etiology of the patient's nausea. If the cause is multifactorial, then multiple agents may be required. Somatostatin analogues should be used in conjunction with other agents when the cause of nausea is malignant bowel obstruction. Corticosteroids should only be added after a failure of other medications in the setting of small bowel obstruction. If a mechanical obstruction is the underlying cause of these symptoms, intestinal

Table 1
Strategies for the management of nausea of different etiologies

Etiology	Drug Class	Drug Example	Receptor	Site of Action
Opioid induced	Butyrephenones	Haloperidol	D2	CTZ
Gastric stasis	Prokinetics	Metoclopramide	D2	Intestinal
		Domperidone		CTZ
Intestinal obstruction or peritoneal irritation	Phenothiazines Antihistamines Anticholinergics	Prochlorperazine Diphenhydramine Hyoscine	D2 H1 ACHm	CTZ Vomiting center Intestinal
Chemotherapy or PONV	5-HT3 Antagonists	Ondansetron	5-HT3	Intestinal CTZ
Late-onset chemotherapy related	NK1 Antagonists	Aprepitant	NK1	Widespread

Abbreviations: 5-HT3, serotonin type 3; ACHm, muscarinic cholinergic; CTZ, chemoreceptor trigger zone; D2, dopamine type 2; H1, histamine type 1; NK1, neurokinin type 1; PONV, postoperative nausea and vomiting.

decompression should be initiated with a nasogastric tube as more definitive surgical or endoscopic interventions are considered.

Cachexia is another symptom frequently present in patients with PC. Cachexia is often very distressing for both patients and their family members. A common response is for family members to try and provide additional nutritional support to combat these symptoms; however, cachexia, by definition, is a failure of nutritional improvement despite adequate protein nutrition. Patients are often unable to tolerate extra nutrition secondary to bowel dysmotility, anorexia, and other associated gastrointestinal symptoms. Efforts to better understand the underlying causes of cachexia and available supportive measures are ongoing. Although nutritional support should be provided, either in enteral or parenteral forms, this modality alone will not resolve cachexia. Supportive care with antiemetics, pain management, pancreatic enzymes, and physical activity should be used based on the underlying cause of patients' inability to tolerate oral intake. Pharmacologic approaches are numerous and include megestrol, ghrelin analogs, cannabinoids, and nonsteroidal anti-inflammatory drugs.[24] The use of medications should be personalized based on the etiology of patients' cachexia, medication side effect profiles, and patient tolerance (**Table 2**). Most medications improve appetite; however, whether or not this strategy leads to improvements in weight or overall nutrition is unclear. All pharmacologic approaches to cachexia require further study to determine their optimal use. One on-going trial is assessing a multimodal treatment approach, including exercise, nutritional education and supplementation, and anti-inflammatory medications.[25]

Fatigue is one of the most severe and bothersome symptoms experienced by patients with advanced cancer.[26] Although fatigue is sometimes related to cachexia, this symptom most likely results from a complex network of etiologies, including the cancer treatments, deconditioning, comorbid medical conditions, and complex psychosocial factors. Fatigue has negative effects on physical, social, and cognitive functioning, and causes distress to patients and their family members.[27] Addressing sleep schedules and poor sleep hygiene is a necessary first step in addressing fatigue. Other nonpharmacologic approaches, such as exercise, education, and assistance with

Table 2
Pharmacologic approaches to the management of cachexia in patients with PC

Medication Class	Benefits	Risks
Anabolic steroids[71]	Appetite stimulant	Less effective than megestrol Not associated with weight gain
Cannabis and cannabinoids (dronabinol)	Appetite stimulant	Possibly decreases quality of life
Glucocorticoids (prednisone, dexamethasone)[72]	Appetite stimulant Improves well-being	Effect short lived Not associated with weight gain Muscle wasting Multiple side effects
Ghrelin analogs[73]	Increases weight Increases lean body mass	Poor quality of evidence No increase in strength
Nonsteroidal anti-inflammatory drugs	Increases weight Improves well-being	Poor quality of evidence
Olanzapine	Increases weight Also treats nausea Few side effects	Poor quality of evidence
Prokinetic agents (metoclopramide, erythromycin)	Improves gastric motility – use when early satiety is cause of cachexia Few side effects	Unknown effect on weight gain
Synthetic progesterone derivates (medroxyprogesterone, megestrol acetate)[74]	Appetite stimulant Small increase in weight	No impact on quality of life Multiple side effects Venous thromboembolism Fluid retention Increased mortality at high doses High cost
Thalidomide[75]	Increases weight Few side effects	No impact on quality of life Poor quality of evidence

changing schedules to lessen fatigue, have been shown to be effective. Acupuncture, yoga, massage, music therapy, and other mindfulness-based approaches have also been shown to improve fatigue significantly.[28,29] Pharmacologic approaches include use of psychostimulants, wakefulness agents, and dietary supplements. The American Society of Clinical Oncology recommends use of psychostimulants (eg, methylphenidate) or wakefulness agents (eg, modafinil) to improve fatigue.[30,31] They can still be effective, but have less impact on fatigue in patients who are not undergoing active treatment. The use of dietary supplements, such as guarana, L-carnitine, and ginseng, have also been studied, although the evidence is mixed and larger studies are needed before these can be recommended routinely.[32] Most therapies for fatigue are low risk and patients should be encouraged to pursue nonpharmacologic therapies. Pharmacologic therapies should be added if these fail or patients suffer from severe symptoms.

These symptoms, particularly cachexia and fatigue, are often accompanied by anhedonia. This situation is often a sign of unrecognized existential distress and warrants consultation with a palliative care and psycho-oncology provider.

MANAGEMENT OF MECHANICAL BOWEL OBSTRUCTIONS FROM A PALLIATIVE CARE PERSPECTIVE
Patient Evaluation Overview

Malignant bowel obstructions related to PC are some of the most challenging complications for providers to manage. Bowel obstructions may arise proximally with gastric outlet or duodenal obstruction, within the small intestine or the proximal colon, or distally in the sigmoid colon and rectum, each with unique characteristics of management (**Fig. 2**). Regardless of the location of obstruction, nonoperative treatment strategies should be considered and discussed with the patients initially, unless the patient has signs or symptoms indicating a need for more urgent operative intervention. These symptoms include clinical signs of peritonitis, hemodynamic instability, or signs of ischemia or perforation on a computed tomography scan, such as free intra-abdominal air or evidence of a closed loop obstruction.

Medical Treatment Options

The initial management should consist of making the patient nil per os, starting appropriate intravenous fluid resuscitation, and correcting metabolic abnormalities, with attention to the patient's medical comorbidities. A nasogastric tube should be placed if the patient is vomiting. An imaging study of the abdomen is necessary to provide diagnostic information on the nature and level of the obstruction, the presence of complications such as bowel ischemia or perforation, and information about the patient's disease state, such as the degree of tumor burden or presence of malignant ascites. Without an obvious need for urgent surgery, patients can usually be monitored carefully. Serial abdominal examinations are imperative in this setting to monitor for signs or symptoms of peritonitis or decompensation. Medical management alone is sometimes successful at alleviating the obstruction, although this approach sometimes requires prolonged periods of enteric rest. Many patients with PC are malnourished before developing an obstruction and early parenteral nutrition should be considered. The American Society for Parenteral and Enteral Nutrition guidelines should be used to determine the degree of malnutrition and need for nutritional support for individual patients.[33] Additionally, all patients should have their symptoms, including pain and nausea, managed aggressively in accordance with the previously noted recommendations.[14]

Surgical and Interventional Treatment Options

A closed loop obstruction, bowel ischemia or perforation, or signs and symptoms of peritonitis are indications to consider urgent operative intervention. Surgery in this

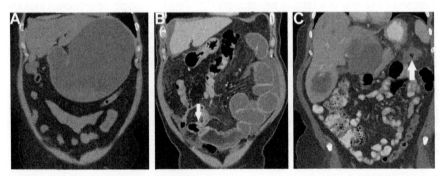

Fig. 2. Cross-sectional imaging demonstrating (A) a proximal obstruction, (B) a midintestinal obstruction, and (C) a distal obstruction from PC.

patient population comes with a relatively high risk of morbidity and mortality, and patient selection is critical. To help determine who would benefit from an operation in this setting, the cooperative group Southwestern Oncology Group (SWOG) is conducting a multicenter, prospective clinical trial randomizing patients to operative and nonoperative management of malignant bowel obstructions for comparison (SWOG S1316).[34] The required operative intervention is often determined at the time of surgery and may consist of a lysis of adhesions, segmental bowel resection, diversion with a loop ostomy or end-ostomy (either small bowel or colon, depending on the obstruction location), or intestinal bypass. If operative resolution of the obstruction cannot be accomplished or would require high-risk surgical procedures, the placement of a gastrostomy tube for venting the stomach can be performed.

Gastric outlet, duodenal, or other proximal obstructions typically present with nausea, vomiting, and upper abdominal distention. During medical management, attention should be paid to repletion of chloride, which is lost with large volume gastric secretion losses. Proximal obstructions are managed similarly to other obstructions initially; however, other definitive treatment options are available for these patients. The placement of a venting gastrostomy tube is often a good option for patients with this pathology, with or without a feeding jejunostomy tube.

Another unique option for gastric outlet obstruction related to PC is intraluminal stenting. Placement of self-expanding metal stents (SEMS) to relieve gastric outlet obstruction has been shown to result in rapid improvement in symptoms, shorter times to oral intake tolerance, and a decreased length of stay compared with open surgical bypass (**Fig. 3**A).[35] SEMS is not without complications, however. Gastric ulceration, iatrogenic perforation, biliary obstruction, stent dysfunction, and stent migration can all occur. SEMS is also much more likely to require repeat intervention than surgical bypass.[36] Patients with multiple sites of obstruction should not undergo SEMS, and patients at high risk for distal obstruction should be approached cautiously when considering SEMS. Although the benefits of SEMS are clear, surgical bypass may also

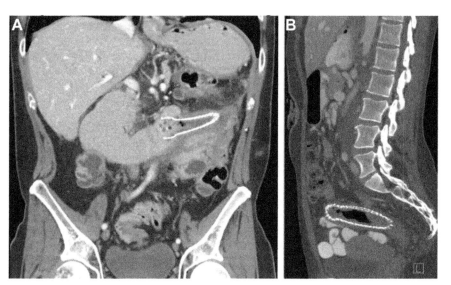

Fig. 3. Cross-sectional imaging of (*A*) a proximal and (*B*) rectal stent placed for the relief of a malignant bowel obstruction related to PC.

be considered. PC is an independent risk factor for mortality after surgical bypass (23.1% vs 6.1%; $P = .046$); however, it remains a valid therapeutic option in appropriately selected patients.[37] Laparoscopic surgical bypass should be attempted if possible, because this approach has been shown to have a lower morbidity and improved functional outcomes compared with an open approach.[38]

Endoscopic stenting is also an option for patients with colonic obstructions (Fig. 3B). PC is a risk factor for technical and clinical failure of stent placement, with the degree of carcinomatosis effecting the likelihood of success.[39,40] Despite this caveat, success rates are high overall, ranging from 63% to 85%.[39,41,42] In patients with good functional status, early clinical success between SEMS and surgery are similar. However, in comparison to surgery, SEMS is associated with higher rates of late adverse events (27.4% vs 9.8%; $P = .005$), decreased patency time (163 vs 349 days; $P<.001$), and an increased need for reintervention (11% vs 2.4% with early reintervention [$P = .153$]; and 26% vs 4.9% for late reintervention [$P = .005$]).[43] Lee and colleagues[44] noted similar findings with high rates of late stent-related complications. SEMS is an excellent option for patients with a severely limited prognosis to avoid a high-risk operation that typically involves intestinal diversion with an ostomy. Like gastric outlet obstructions related to PC, a patient's preoperative nutritional status and functional status should be taken into account when considering endoscopic stenting versus surgery.

PALLIATIVE MANAGEMENT OF FISTULAE

Another complication encountered by patients with PC is the development of fistulae from the bowel to the skin or other organs. This complication may be the result of the tumor itself or a complication of treatment. Enterocutaneous fistulas occur in 4% to 34% of patients after cytoreductive surgery for PC.[45] Fistulae are most often formed between the bowel and the bladder, uterus, or vagina, but sometimes involve other adjacent organs, including the ovaries and ureters. This development is a particularly difficult challenge because fistulae often occur in areas where patients have had prior surgery or radiation. Optimal palliative management must be individualized based on the patient's underlying prognosis and overall health status, as well as the anatomy of the fistulae and symptomatology. Cross-sectional imaging (computed tomography scans and MRI) is superior to fluoroscopic imaging for evaluating fistulae, and should be performed before developing an individualized treatment strategy; however, a combination of imaging techniques is often required to define the exact location, size, and complexity of the fistula.[46]

Palliative therapies for pelvic fistulae range from simple drainage procedures, such as urinary drainage for a vesicovaginal fistula, to total pelvic exenteration for an isolated pelvic tumor with severe life-limiting symptoms. Complex cases should be managed by a surgical oncologist-led multidisciplinary team including gynecologic oncologists, urologists, and plastic and reconstructive surgeons as needed. Before undertaking the large abdominal operations often required for resolution of fistulae, such as pelvic exenteration, diagnostic laparoscopy can be helpful to ensure that the actual burden of peritoneal disease is consistent with what is demonstrated on imaging.[47] Computed tomography imaging accurately depicts the extent of disease in 60% of patients, but can underestimate the size of lesions in up to 33%.[48] Other surgical options include endoscopically or fluoroscopically placed stents, or diversion—either intestinal (ileostomy or colostomy) or urinary (nephrostomy or cystostomy). Data on patient-centered outcomes are lacking with regard to patient acceptance of diverting ostomies for palliative therapy. However, diversion can often lead to improvements in quality of life by decreasing pain, improving nutrition, or allowing for the receipt of additional palliative chemotherapy, and should be considered a valid treatment option.

MANAGEMENT OF MALIGNANT ASCITES FROM A PALLIATIVE CARE PERSPECTIVE

Malignant ascites also occurs frequently in patients with PC. Malignant ascites is a poor prognostic indicator, with a median survival of less than 6 months from the time of ascites development.[49] Malignant ascites and its associated symptoms (pain, nausea, dyspnea, and anorexia) can greatly decrease patients' quality of life. Decreasing the quantity of the ascites can help to palliate many of these symptoms. The medical management of malignant ascites, through sodium restriction and diuretics, is effective in only 22% to 40% of patients.[49] If attempted, diuretics should be used with caution, because dehydration and electrolyte abnormalities from this treatment are common.

Paracentesis offers rapid relief of symptoms from malignant ascites and should be used as first-line therapy for most patients. Unfortunately, symptoms return rapidly, typically within 48 to 72 hours. If patients require multiple repeat paracenteses or have a rapid return of symptoms from ascites after treatment, indwelling tunneled catheters are another effective palliative option. Nontunneled catheters have also been used, but are associated with higher complication rates, including both cellulitis and intra-abdominal infections. Nontunneled catheters should be avoided in all patients except those with a very limited prognosis, with life expectancy measured in weeks. Tunneled catheters can be placed under local anesthesia by surgery or interventional radiology. Complications from tunneled catheters are rare, and the vast majority significantly improve quality of life and remain in place and functioning for the remainder of the patient's life.[50,51] These devices can be connected intermittently to a self-contained vacuum drainage system at home, preventing the need for frequent hospital visits. Intraperitoneal ports are also an effective, durable option for patients with refractory ascites.[52] Peritonovenous shunts have also been used for treatment of malignant ascites; however, the effectiveness is lower and the complication rate is higher than the interventional options mentioned elsewhere in this article.[53]

Hyperthermic intraperitoneal chemoperfusion is another effective option for management of malignant ascites (**Table 3**).[54–63] Although sometimes requiring multiple treatments, hyperthermic intraperitoneal chemoperfusion can be delivered in a minimally invasive fashion via laparoscopy or even with only ultrasound guidance.[57,61] Once the catheters are in place, subsequent treatments can be performed in an intensive care unit.

With multiple procedural options for ascites management, providers must consider an individual patient's functional status and overall prognosis when deciding on the best palliative intervention. With poor functional status and severely limited life expectancy, repeat paracentesis is likely the best palliative option. With life expectancy measured in weeks or months, indwelling catheters or ports are a good option. Hyperthermic intraperitoneal chemoperfusion should be considered for patients with a relatively improved functional status and longer life expectancy, because this therapy is associated with more adverse events than repeated drainage.

Often, other complications of PC present in patients with malignant ascites. In patients with malignant bowel obstructions or bowel dysmotility, clinicians are often reluctant to offer interventional solutions. Surgical outcomes in patients with malignant ascites are poor and are accompanied by higher rates of morbidity and mortality. Malignant ascites also raises concerns of an increased risk of infectious complications related to spillage of enteric contents into the ascites and poor wound healing of the abdominal wall secondary to leakage of ascites. Despite these theoretic risks,

Table 3
Outcomes of palliative HIPEC for the management of malignant ascites related to PC

Author, Year	N	Tumor	Agent(s)	Technique	Response (%)	Median Survival
Jiao et al,[63] 2020	45	Varied	Varied	Laparoscopic	91	N/A
Orgiano et al,[58] 2016	15	Varied	Varied	Bedside catheter placement	100	N/A
Valle et al,[54] 2015	12	Varied	Varied	Laparoscopic	83	57 d
Randle et al,[62] 2014	299	Varied	Varied	Open, with CRS	93	5.6 mo[a]
Ba et al,[57] 2013	62	Ovarian	Cisplatin and doxorubicin	Laparoscopic or B-ultrasound guided	93	8 mo (2–20)
		Gastrointestinal	Mitomycin	B-ultrasound guided	94	9 mo (2–30)
Cui et al,[61] 2012	32	Varied	Cisplatin and doxorubicin or mitomycin	B-ultrasound guided	94	9 mo
Valle et al,[55] 2009	52	Varied	Cisplatin and doxorubicin or mitomycin	Laparoscopic	98	98 d (21–796)
Facchiano et al,[59] 2008	5	Gastric	Mitomycin and cisplatin	Laparoscopic	100	89 d (33–144)
Garofalo et al,[60] 2006	14	Varied	Cisplatin and doxorubicin or mitomycin	Laparoscopic	100	203 d (21–667)

Abbreviations: CRS, cytoreductive surgery; HIPEC, hyperthermic intraperitoneal chemotherapy; N/A, not applicable.
[a] Median survival for patients with incomplete CRS only.

placement of a decompressive gastrostomy tube has been shown to be a good option for these patients. Although the complication rates are relatively high (9%–36%), the procedure can be performed successfully in the majority of patients.[64,65] Many complications are related to tube malfunction or the need for reintervention, and not the more feared gastric leak and subsequent intra-abdominal infection. Paracentesis, or the concurrent placement of a tunneled peritoneal catheter, is advised.

PALLIATIVE SURGERY: THE IMPORTANCE OF PATIENT SELECTION

The decision to proceed with a surgical intervention for palliation at the end of life presents a major challenge to patients and health care providers. In patients with PC, an emergent operation can rescue patients from a life-threatening complication, even though the surgery is not aimed at curing the patient of their underlying disease. These situations are emotionally charged and highly stressful for patients, family members, and providers.

Emergent surgery in patients with PC often bears a relatively higher risk than similar surgery in patients without PC. Although most patients survive the initial operation, many die soon after surgery and the majority experience postoperative complications, a need for reoperation, nursing home stays, and/or hospital readmissions.[26] Cauley and colleagues[66] reported the results of a retrospective study analyzing outcomes of patients with disseminated cancer undergoing emergency surgery (376 for obstruction and 499 for perforation). Operations for perforation resulted in a 30-day mortality rate of 34% and morbidity rate of 67%, with 52% of patients discharged to an institution. Operations for obstruction resulted in a 30-day mortality rate of 18% and a morbidity rate of 41%, with 60% of patients discharged to an institution. Other studies have noted similar outcomes.[67,68] Even with successful initial management, reobstruction (6%–47%), reoperation (2%–15%), and readmission rates (38%–74%) are high.[69] Patients who do undergo surgery often spend a high number of their remaining days (6%–61%) in the hospital.[69,70] Oral intake after surgery is only possible in 45% to 75% of patients.[69] It is incumbent upon the surgical provider to adequately and sensitively inform patients of these risks, including setting realistic expectations for the postoperative experience and expected quality of life. Further study is needed to better understand patients' quality of life after palliative surgical intervention in the setting of advanced malignancy.

Dependent functional status, older age, the presence of ascites, and preoperative nutritional status are associated with poorer operative outcomes after emergent and palliative procedures.[66,67,70] These factors should all be considered in operative decision-making. The challenges demonstrated by these data require surgeons and other providers to set realistic expectations for patients and their families. Despite the knowledge of the presence of a life-limiting condition, many people are still not prepared to die when a life-threatening surgical complication occurs. Many, regardless of the potential challenges posed by surgery, are willing to undertake any risk to prolong life. Unfortunately, no specific guidelines exist regarding the role of surgery in this setting and providers and patients must rely on the experience and expertise of the involved surgeons. Therefore, early involvement of palliative care and ACP are essential during these stressful scenarios to help patients with decision-making and the possible transition into end-of-life care.

SUMMARY

PC is associated with myriad symptoms that negatively impact patients' quality of life. Complications related to PC, including malignant bowel obstructions and malignant ascites, are some of the most challenging problems for both patients and their health care providers. Numerous medical, interventional, and surgical treatment options exist to help alleviate the suffering caused by PC. Providing the optimal treatment for individual patients must take into account patient preferences, patient functional and nutritional status, and the overall prognosis. The early involvement of palliative care within a multidisciplinary care team is essential to provide patients with optimal, holistic care.

CLINICS CARE POINTS

- Early involvement of a palliative care team is essential to providing optimal, holistic care to patients with PC.
- Symptoms of pain, nausea, cachexia, and fatigue are very common with PC and should be treated aggressively.
- Multiple options are available to treat complications of PC, including malignant bowel obstructions or malignant ascites, and treatment choices should reflect individual patient desires and disease characteristics.
- Although surgical intervention in patients with PC can be high risk, operative interventions can provide excellent palliative management in appropriately selected patients.
- Heated intraperitoneal chemotherapy should be considered for management of refractory malignant ascites in patients with PC.

DISCLOSURE

The authors have nothing to disclose.

REFERENCES

1. Miller J, Wynn WH. A malignant tumour arising from the endothelium of the peritoneum, and producing a mucoid ascitic fluid. J Pathol Bacteriol 1908;12(2):267–78.
2. National Comprehensive Cancer Network. Palliative Care. Vol 1; 2020.
3. Ferrell BR, Temel JS, Temin S, et al. Integration of palliative care into standard oncology care: American Society of Clinical Oncology clinical practice guideline update. J Clin Oncol 2017;35(1):96–112.
4. Plana A, Izquierdo FJ, Schuitevoerder D, et al. The Chicago Consensus on peritoneal surface malignancies: palliative care considerations. Ann Surg Oncol 2020;27(6):1798–804.
5. Plana A, Izquierdo FJ, Schuitevoerder D, et al. The Chicago Consensus on peritoneal surface malignancies: standards. Ann Surg Oncol 2020;27(6):1743–52.
6. Hawley PH. The bow tie model of 21st century palliative care. J Pain Symptom Manage 2014;47(1):2–5.
7. Barnato AE. Challenges in understanding and respecting patients' preferences. Health Aff 2017;36(7):1252–7.
8. Sudore RL. Redefining the "Planning" in advance care planning: preparing for end-of-life decision making. Ann Intern Med 2010;153(4):256.
9. Levoy K, Buck H, Behar-Zusman V. The impact of varying levels of advance care planning engagement on perceptions of the end-of-life experience among caregivers of deceased patients with cancer. Am J Hosp Palliat Med 2020. https://doi.org/10.1177/1049909120917899.

10. Bischoff KE, Sudore R, Miao Y, et al. Advance care planning and the quality of end-of-life care in older adults. J Am Geriatr Soc 2013;61(2):209–14.

11. Magge D, Zenati MS, Austin F, et al. Malignant peritoneal mesothelioma: prognostic factors and oncologic outcome analysis. Ann Surg Oncol 2014;21(4): 1159–65.

12. Pletcher E, Gleeson E, Labow D. Peritoneal cancers and hyperthermic intraperitoneal chemotherapy. Surg Clin North Am 2020;100(3):589–613.

13. Goff BA, Mandel LS, Melancon CH, et al. Frequency of symptoms of ovarian cancer in women presenting to primary care clinics. J Am Med Assoc 2004;291(22): 2705–12.

14. World Health Organization. WHO's cancer pain ladder for adults 1986. p. 1–2. Available at: http://www.who.int/cancer/palliative/painladder/en/. Accessed December 20, 2020.

15. Anekar AA, Cascella M. WHO Analgesic Ladder. In: StatPearls [Internet]. Treasure Island (FL): StatPearls Publishing; 2020. p. 1–10. Available at: https://www.ncbi.nlm.nih.gov/books/NBK554435/#_NBK554435_pubdet_.

16. Cuomo A, Bimonte S, Forte CA, et al. Multimodal approaches and tailored therapies for pain management: the trolley analgesic model. J Pain Res 2019;12: 711–4.

17. Laval G, Marcelin-Benazech B, Guirimand F, et al. Recommendations for bowel obstruction with peritoneal carcinomatosis. J Pain Symptom Manage 2014; 48(1):75–91.

18. Wickham RJ. Nausea and vomiting: a palliative care imperative. Curr Oncol Rep 2020;22(1). https://doi.org/10.1007/s11912-020-0871-6.

19. Peng X, Wang P, Li S, et al. Randomized clinical trial comparing octreotide and scopolamine butylbromide in symptom control of patients with inoperable bowel obstruction due to advanced ovarian cancer. World J Surg Oncol 2015;13(1):1–6.

20. Mariani P, Blumberg J, Landau A, et al. Symptomatic treatment with lanreotide microparticles in inoperable bowel obstruction resulting from peritoneal carcinomatosis: a randomized, double-blind, placebo-controlled phase III study. J Clin Oncol 2012;30(35):4337–43.

21. Minoura T, Takeuchi M, Morita T, et al. Practice patterns of medications for patients with malignant bowel obstruction using a nationwide claims database and the association between treatment outcomes and concomitant use of H2-blockers/proton pump inhibitors and corticosteroids with octreotide. J Pain Symptom Manage 2018;55(2):413–9.e2.

22. Feuer D, Broadley K. Surgery for the resolution of symptoms in malignant bowel obstruction in advanced gynaecological and gastrointestinal cancer (Review). Cochrane Database Syst Rev 2000;3. https://doi.org/10.1002/14651858. CD002764.pub2.

23. Clark K, Lam L, Currow D. Reducing gastric secretions - a role for histamine 2 antagonists or proton pump inhibitors in malignant bowel obstruction? Support Care Cancer 2009;17(12):1463–8.

24. Ohnuma T, Ali M, Adigun R. Supportive Care in Cancer Therapy: Anorexia and Cachexia. Humana Press; September 2008.pp. 47-86. http://doi.org/10.1007/978-1-59745-291-5_4.

25. Solheim TS, Laird BJA, Balstad TR, et al. Cancer cachexia: rationale for the MENAC (Multimodal - Exercise, Nutrition and Anti-inflammatory medication for Cachexia) trial. BMJ Support Palliat Care 2018;258–65. https://doi.org/10.1136/bmjspcare-2017-001440.

26. Li B, Mah K, Swami N, et al. Symptom assessment in patients with advanced cancer: are the most severe symptoms the most bothersome? J Palliat Med 2019; 22(10):1252–9.

27. Mitchell SA, Hoffman AJ, Clark JC, et al. Putting evidence into practice: an update of evidence-based interventions for cancer-related fatigue during and following treatment. Clin J Oncol Nurs 2014;18(6):38–58.

28. Jacobsen PB, Donovan KA, Vadaparampil ST, et al. Systematic review and meta-analysis of psychological and activity-based interventions for cancer-related fatigue. Heal Psychol 2007;26(6):660–7.

29. Sood A, Barton DL, Bauer BA, et al. A critical review of complementary therapies for cancer-related fatigue. Integr Cancer Ther 2007;6(1):8–13.

30. Bower JE, Bak K, Berger A, et al. Screening, assessment, and management of fatigue in adult survivors of cancer: an American Society of Clinical Oncology clinical practice guideline adaptation. J Clin Oncol 2014;32(17):1840–50.

31. Qu D, Zhang Z, Yu X, et al. Psychotropic drugs for the management of cancer-related fatigue: a systematic review and meta-analysis. Eur J Cancer Care (Engl) 2016;25(6):970–9.

32. National Comprehensive Cancer Network. Cancer-Related Fatigue: NCCN Clinical Practice Guidelines in Oncology; 2020.

33. Mueller C, Compher C, Ellen DM. A.S.P.E.N. clinical guidelines: nutrition screening, assessment, and intervention in adults. J Parenter Enter Nutr 2011; 35(1):16–24.

34. SWOG: Cancer Research Network. SWOG study S1316 page 2020. Available at: https://www.swog.org/swog-study-s1316-page. Accessed December 20, 2020.

35. Ly J, O'Grady G, Mittal A, et al. A systematic review of methods to palliate malignant gastric outlet obstruction. Surg Endosc 2010;24(2):290–7.

36. Mintziras I, Miligkos M, Wächter S, et al. Palliative surgical bypass is superior to palliative endoscopic stenting in patients with malignant gastric outlet obstruction: systematic review and meta-analysis. Surg Endosc 2019;33(10):3153–64.

37. Bednarsch J, Czigany Z, Heise D, et al. Influence of peritoneal carcinomatosis on perioperative outcome in palliative gastric bypass for malignant gastric outlet obstruction- A retrospective cohort study. World J Surg Oncol 2020;18(1):1–8.

38. Ojima T, Nakamori M, Nakamura M, et al. Laparoscopic gastrojejunostomy for patients with unresectable gastric cancer with gastric outlet obstruction. J Gastrointest Surg 2017;21(8):1220–5.

39. Park JJ, Rhee K, Yoon JY, et al. Impact of peritoneal carcinomatosis on clinical outcomes of patients receiving self-expandable metal stents for malignant colorectal obstruction. Endoscopy 2018;50(12):1163–74.

40. Kuwai T, Yamaguchi T, Imagawa H, et al. Factors related to difficult self-expandable metallic stent placement for malignant colonic obstruction: a post-hoc analysis of a multicenter study across Japan. Dig Endosc 2019;31(1):51–8.

41. Kim JH, Ku YS, Jeon TJ, et al. The efficacy of self-expanding metal stents for malignant colorectal obstruction by noncolonic malignancy with peritoneal carcinomatosis. Dis Colon Rectum 2013;56(11):1228–32.

42. Caceres A, Zhou Q, Iasonos A, et al. Colorectal stents for palliation of large-bowel obstructions in recurrent gynecologic cancer: an updated series. Gynecol Oncol 2008;108(3):482–5.

43. Ahn HJ, Kim SW, Lee SW, et al. Long-term outcomes of palliation for unresectable colorectal cancer obstruction in patients with good performance status: endoscopic stent versus surgery. Surg Endosc 2016;30(11):4765–75.

44. Lee HJ, Park SJ, Min BS, et al. The role of primary colectomy after successful endoscopic stenting in patients with obstructive metastatic colorectal cancer. Dis Colon Rectum 2014;57(6):694–9.

45. Valle SJ, Alzahrani N, Alzahrani S, et al. Enterocutaneous fistula in patients with peritoneal malignancy following cytoreductive surgery and hyperthermic intraperitoneal chemotherapy: incidence, management and outcomes. Surg Oncol 2016; 25(3):315–20.

46. Narayanan P, Reznek RH, Andrea Rockall MbbcG. Fistulas in malignant gynecologic disease: etiology, imaging, and management. RadioGraphics 2009;29: 1073–84.

47. Rivard JD, Temple WJ, McConnell YJ, et al. Preoperative computed tomography does not predict resectability in peritoneal carcinomatosis. Am J Surg 2014; 207(5):760–5.

48. Koh JL, Yan TD, Glenn D, et al. Evaluation of preoperative computed tomography in estimating peritoneal cancer index in colorectal peritoneal carcinomatosis. Ann Surg Oncol 2009;16(2):327–33.

49. Hodge C, Badgwell BD. Palliation of malignant ascites. J Surg Oncol 2019; 120(1):67–73.

50. Wong BCT, Cake L, Kachuik L, et al. Indwelling peritoneal catheters for managing malignancy-associated ascites. J Palliat Care 2015;31(4):243–9.

51. Knight JA, Thompson SM, Fleming CJ, et al. Safety and effectiveness of palliative tunneled peritoneal drainage catheters in the management of refractory malignant and non-malignant ascites. Cardiovasc Intervent Radiol 2018;41(5):753–61.

52. Coupe NA, Cox K, Clark K, et al. Outcomes of permanent peritoneal ports for the management of recurrent malignant ascites. J Palliat Med 2013;16(8):938–40.

53. Stukan M. Drainage of malignant ascites: patient selection and perspectives. Cancer Manag Res 2017;9:115–30.

54. Valle SJ, Alzahrani NA, Alzahrani SE, et al. Laparoscopic hyperthermic intraperitoneal chemotherapy (HIPEC) for refractory malignant ascites in patients unsuitable for cytoreductive surgery. Int J Surg 2015;23:176–80.

55. Valle M, Van Der Speeten K, Garofalo A. Laparoscopic hyperthermic intraperitoneal peroperative chemotherapy (HIPEC) in the management of refractory malignant ascites: a multi-institutional retrospective analysis in 52 patients. J Surg Oncol 2009;100(4):331–4.

56. Ba M, Long H, Zhang X, et al. Hyperthermic intraperitoneal perfusion chemotherapy and cytoreductive surgery for controlling malignant ascites from ovarian cancer. Int J Gynecol Cancer 2016;26(9):1571–9.

57. Ba MC, Long H, Cui SZ, et al. Multivariate comparison of B-ultrasound guided and laparoscopic continuous circulatory hyperthermic intraperitoneal perfusion chemotherapy for malignant ascites. Surg Endosc 2013;27(8):2735–43.

58. Orgiano L, Pani F, Astara G, et al. The role of "closed abdomen" hyperthermic intraperitoneal chemotherapy (HIPEC) in the palliative treatment of neoplastic ascites from peritoneal carcinomatosis: report of a single-center experience. Support Care Cancer 2016;24(10):4293–9.

59. Facchiano E, Scaringi S, Kianmanesh R, et al. Laparoscopic hyperthermic intraperitoneal chemotherapy (HIPEC) for the treatment of malignant ascites secondary to unresectable peritoneal carcinomatosis from advanced gastric cancer. Eur J Surg Oncol 2008;34(2):154–8.

60. Garofalo A, Valle M, Garcia J, et al. Laparoscopic intraperitoneal hyperthermic chemotherapy for palliation of debilitating malignant ascites. Eur J Surg Oncol 2006;32(6):682–5.

61. Cui S, Ba M, Tang Y, et al. B ultrasound-guided hyperthermic intraperitoneal perfusion chemotherapy for the treatment of malignant ascites. Oncol Rep 2012;28(4):1325–31.

62. Randle RW, Swett KR, Swords DS, et al. Efficacy of cytoreductive surgery with hyperthermic intraperitoneal chemotherapy in the management of malignant ascites. Ann Surg Oncol 2014;21(5):1474–9.

63. Jiao J, Li C, Yu G, et al. Efficacy of hyperthermic intraperitoneal chemotherapy (HIPEC) in the management of malignant ascites. World J Surg Oncol 2020; 18(1):1–6.

64. O'connor OJ, Diver E, Mcdermott S, et al. Palliative gastrostomy in the setting of voluminous ascites. J Palliat Med 2014;17(7):811–21.

65. Shaw C, Bassett RL, Fox PS, et al. Palliative venting gastrostomy in patients with malignant bowel obstruction and ascites. Ann Surg Oncol 2013;20(2):497–505.

66. Cauley CE, Panizales MT, Reznor G, et al. Outcomes after emergency abdominal surgery in patients with advanced cancer. J Trauma Acute Care Surg 2015;79(3): 399–406.

67. Cousins S, Tempest E, Feuer DJ. Surgery for the resolution of symptoms in malignant bowel obstruction in advanced gynaecological and gastrointestinal cancer (Cochrane Review). Cochrane Database Syst Rev 2000;4(1). https://doi.org/10.1002/14651858.CD002764.pub2.

68. Bento de JH, Bianchi ET, Tustumi F, et al. Surgical management of malignant intestinal obstruction: outcome and prognostic factors. Chirurgia (Bucur) 2019; 114(3):343.

69. Olson TJP, Pinkerton C, Brasel KJ, et al. Palliative surgery for malignant bowel obstruction from carcinomatosis a systematic review. JAMA Surg 2014;149(4): 383–92.

70. Blair SL, Chu DZJ, Schwarz RE. Outcome of palliative operations for malignant bowel obstruction in patients with peritoneal carcinomatosis from nongynecological cancer. Ann Surg Oncol 2001;8(8):632–7.

71. Loprinzi BCL, Kugler JW, Sloan JA, et al. Randomized comparison of megestrol acetate versus dexamethasone versus fluoxymesterone for the treatment of cancer anorexia/cachexia. J Clin Oncol 1999;17(10):3299–306.

72. Miller S, McNutt L, McCann MA, et al. Use of corticosteroids for anorexia in palliative medicine: a systematic review. J Palliat Med 2014;17(4):482–5.

73. Malik JS, Yennurajalingam S. Prokinetics and ghrelin for the management of cancer cachexia syndrome. Ann Palliat Med 2019;8(1):80–5.

74. Ruiz Garcia V, López-Briz E, Carbonell Sanchis R, et al. Megestrol acetate for treatment of anorexia-cachexia syndrome. Cochrane Database Syst Rev 2013; 2017(7). https://doi.org/10.1002/14651858.CD004310.pub3.

75. Gordon JN, Trebble TM, Ellis RD, et al. Thalidomide in the treatment of cancer cachexia: a randomised placebo controlled trial. Gut 2005;54(4):540–5.

Evaluation and Management of Malignant Biliary Obstruction

Nadia V. Guardado, MD[a], Kaysey Llorente, MD[a],
Benoit Blondeau, MD, MBA[b,c],*

KEYWORDS

- Biliary malignancies • Malignant obstructive jaundice • Surgical palliative care
- Futility of care • Difficult conversation

KEY POINTS

- Conditions causing malignant biliary obstruction evolve silently and appear often at advanced stages.
- Imaging has optimized staging and decompression.
- Endoluminal techniques have replaced, when available, surgical procedures for palliation.
- Still a set of rapidly deadly diseases.
- Supportive and palliative care often are not available.

INTRODUCTION AND HISTORICAL PERSPECTIVE

Surgical intervention was the only option for the management of patients affected by malignant biliary obstruction (MBO), both for curative intent and for symptom management, for decades. Even in the most optimal presentation, midterm survival was mediocre at best, and long-term survival anecdotal. Realism and decency guided the management of this subset of aggressive cancers by surgical pioneers until the 1970s. Surgical palliation was piloted by intraoperative staging and symptom management because curative intention rarely was attainable. Currently, palliation still is the main philosophy for the management of many patients given the advanced stage at presentation and associated limited life expectancy.

[a] Department of Surgery, University of New Mexico School of Medicine, 2425 Camino de Salud, Albuquerque, NM 87106, USA; [b] Department of Surgery, Division of Trauma Surgery, University of New Mexico; [c] Division of Palliative Medicine, University of New Mexico, Albuquerque, NM, USA
* Corresponding author. Department of Surgery, University of New Mexico School of Medicine, University of New Mexico, MSC 10 5610, Albuquerque, NM 87131-0001.
E-mail address: bblondeau@salud.unm.edu
Twitter: @palliativist (B.B.)

Surg Oncol Clin N Am 30 (2021) 491–503
https://doi.org/10.1016/j.soc.2021.03.001
1055-3207/21/© 2021 Elsevier Inc. All rights reserved.

surgonc.theclinics.com

The evolution of death perception over the past 50 years in the United States and the rise of sophisticated and aggressive care has affected the role of palliative care as a valid, equivalent, therapeutic modality for patients affected with deadly conditions. Arguably, society at large benefited from the progress of knowledge, technology, and innovation through the development of aggressive care, occupying a preponderant therapeutic place. This is an industrialized world statement, solipsistic, focused on a small subset of humanity. Most people do not, and never may, have access to the technology described in this article.

The normative concept of life prolongation as the only valid option over patients' choice and quality of life has relegated palliative care to a set of second order measures, with an associated semantic focused on failure and abandonment. The almost singular focus on aggressive care appears to be shifting gradually as increased attention and discussion focuses on patient-centric care. The patient, rather than the medical or scientific community, as definer of beneficial and nonbeneficial therapy is assuming a larger role in the scientific and lay literature. One of the most approachable examples from recent literature is *Being Mortal* by Dr Atul Gawande, a multi-awarded book on the topic of quality of life when quantity no longer is available.[1]

The curability, life expectancy, and quality of life of patients affected by MBO have improved and the once surgical only option has become a complex multimodal catalog of options dedicated to cure and also to improving the symptoms of noncurable patients with longer survival.

The patient's choice is regaining a place that technology has suppressed for a few decades, because the value of life at any cost was, and still might be, the only metric used to gauge efficacy of medical interventions. The multimodal options available in MBO are valid only for the fortunate few who live in a supportive health care system, operationally, financially, and socially. For the others, the immense majority, outcomes might not have changed. Multidisciplinary management requires access to care and there is no causality between level of industrialization and development and universal access to care.

TWO ERAS OF MANAGEMENT

This article is not a systematic review of MBO but a narrative one, because only articles in English and French were reviewed. The literature reviewed is time sensitive and can be separated in 2 different eras, still overlapping, depending on the geographic site of practice of the investigators. The first era starts when surgical intervention was the only option for diagnosis and symptom management; sometimes cure was attainable. The natural history was rapid progression to death within a few months. This still is the decision tree used in many areas of the world. The second era started with the appearance of multimodal therapies and the prospect for improved survival, if not cure. The consequence, intended or not, of this second era of management, has been a transition from individual, patient-centered care toward a focus on aggregated, population-based outcomes (eg, overall survival and progression-free survival). Similarly, the insidious shift in focus from the patient as the center of care and ultimate arbiter of a "good outcome" to a time of aggregate survival also is seen in the language. Cancer patients now can be classified as survivors or not.[2] The corollary is the ranking of the therapeutic options and the race for life at any cost, because only days or weeks count. When population-based outcomes take primacy in determining the benefits of treatment, this also introduces the risk to more vulnerable populations, such as the elderly, who may not experience the same benefits extrapolated from clinical trials of predominantly younger patients.[3] Clear advances of this second era are the development and refinement of alternate modes of technical palliation that certainly have contributed to the improved symptomatic management of this population.[4,5]

APPROACH TO THE JAUNDICE PATIENT

Jaundice is a rare clinical sign in the adult population. In a 2-year study of a family practice patients' cohort, 277 patients of 186,814 (approximately 0.15%) adults older than 45 developed at least 1 episode of jaundice[6]; 33% had bile duct stones, 12% had pancreatic cancer, 5% had cholangiocarcinoma, 10% had another malignancy, and 9% had liver disease. Almost one-quarter, 22%, did not have a record of the diagnosis. As illustrated by these data, the critical need to rule out malignancy as a cause of jaundice not always is appreciated. Furthermore, the urgency of securing a diagnosis is paramount given the aggressive biology of these malignancies.[7] Disparities in access to advanced care, such as endoscopic retrograde cholangiopancreatography (ERCP) in some geographic areas of the United States, and for some ethnic groups also contribute to health care disparities seen in patients with jaundice and the associated underlying malignancies.

By either extrinsic compression or intrinsic formation, biliary obstruction, and the resultant jaundice, often is the initial presenting sign of several hepato-pancreatico-biliary malignancies, as in the classic presentation of jaundice in pancreatic head adenocarcinoma and cholangiocarcinoma. Data from the American Cancer Society published in 2020 reported that pancreatic ductal adenocarcinoma is the fourth leading cause of cancer death in the United States despite its relatively low incidence of approximately 57,600 cases yearly and 47.050 deaths.[8] Approximately 80% of these patients presented with biliary obstruction, typically located at the head of the pancreas or at the uncinate process. As one of the deadliest cancers, the survival rate for patients with advanced pancreatic cancer across all genders and races is approximately 3% at 5 years.[9] Cholangiocarcinoma, although less prevalent, also is a deadly disease; 42,030 cases and 31,780 deaths were reported in 2020.[8] Classified by anatomic location—intrahepatic, perihilar, or distal—cholangiocarcinoma rarely is diagnosed at an early stage. It has an incidence of 1.6 per 100,000 people each year in the United States. Several studies have shown, however, an increased incidence of cholangiocarcinoma over the past decade. The 5-year survival rate for cholangiocarcinoma diagnosed at an advanced stage is approximately 2%.[10]

Although patient history and physical examination are required elements toward making a diagnosis of benign or MBO, advanced imaging and the pathologic evaluation of tissue are mandatory when a malignancy is suspected (discussed later). Classic painless jaundice, the pathognomonic sign of pancreatic head adenocarcinoma, often is associated with nonspecific signs secondary to the systemic effects of biliary retention, including, pruritus, dark urine, and discolored stools, which almost always are present.[11] Important signs for the diagnosis and the prognosis of patients with suspected pancreatic cancer are the presence of unintentional weight loss and new-onset diabetes in an older adult; these findings should be identified as paraneoplastic syndromes associated with pancreatic cancer.[12] Similarly, depression and fatigue may precede the diagnosis.[13] Elevated conjugated bilirubin and alkaline phosphatase are common but nondiagnostic for malignancy. The tumor markers commonly evaluated in patients with biliary obstruction have variable sensitivity and specificity for malignancy. For instance, carbohydrate antigen 19-9 greater than 37 U/mL has a sensitivity of 70% to 86% and specificity of 8% to 90% for MBO whereas carcinoembryonic antigen has a sensitivity of 33% to 68% and a specificity of 75% to 95% for cholangiocarcinoma.[14–16] Recent studies show several other potential tumor markers, including PAM4, glypican 1, KRAS mutations, and microRNAs (miRNAs) used in the early diagnosis of pancreatic cancer. Elevated levels of miRNA-143 and miRNA-30e have a reported sensitivity of 83% and a specificity of 96% for identifying pancreatic cancer.[17]

DIAGNOSIS AND STAGING

The second era of evaluation and management of MBO is characterized by advanced imaging. Although an exhaustive review of pancreaticobiliary imaging is beyond the scope of this article, several key imaging modalities now are used routinely to evaluate patients with MBO. Transabdominal ultrasonography (TAUS) or screening computed tomography (CT) guides the need for further imaging. In many instances, when the findings of these initial imaging studies raise suspicion for a malignant cause of biliary obstruction, referral often is made to a tertiary center where several modalities using various CT scan protocols or magnetic resonance imaging (MRI) or magnetic resonance cholangiopancreatography are used in conjunction with endoluminal procedures to identify lesions, obtain tissue for biopsy, and perform biliary decompression with ERCP. In patients without endoluminal access for biliary decompression or following unsuccessful attempt at endoscopic decompression, percutaneous catheterization of the biliary system by interventional radiology often is required. In a recent systematic review, Toft and colleagues[18] compared sensitivities, specificities, and diagnostic accuracy of several modalities for the diagnosis of pancreatic adenocarcinomas. Sensitivities range from 88% for TAUS to 93% for MRI. Specificity was highest with TAUS at 94% compared with CT with 87%. Finally, accuracy ranged from 89% for CT and endoscopic ultrasound (EUS) to 90% and 91% for MRI and TAUS, respectively.[18]

Confirmation of the diagnosis of malignancy requires pathologic evaluation of tissue, typically obtained through nonsurgical techniques. The combination of EUS and fine-needle aspiration has a high accuracy (93%) for diagnosing pancreatic adenocarcinoma.[19] Mallery and colleagues[20] reported the equivalence of accuracy between EUS, CT scan–guided and surgically obtained biopsies.

TECHNICAL INTERVENTIONS FOR MALIGNANT BILIARY OBSTRUCTION
Surgical Approach

When only surgical procedures were available for evaluation and management of MBO (first era), the techniques dedicated to palliation included cholecystogastrostomy, hepaticojejunostomy, cholecystojejunostomy, and choledochoduodenostomy.[21,22] More recently, Saldinger and colleagues[23] described 2 approaches to palliation of MBO in patients with hilar cholangiocarcinoma. Patients diagnosed with unresectable tumors preoperatively are offered percutaneous drainage whereas those determined to be unresectable intraoperatively undergo biliointestinal bypass. Palliative surgery proportionally has decreased with the advent of improved preoperative imaging and interventional procedures. **Fig. 1** shows an algorithm with currently available therapy options to help guide treatment of symptomatic relief of MBO.

Endoluminal and Percutaneous Therapies

The major procedural change in the management of MBO is the shift from open surgical procedures to percutaneous and endoluminal interventions, at the end of the 1970s.[24] The time when laparotomy was required for staging and palliative bypass largely has passed. Endoluminal and percutaneous techniques have variable

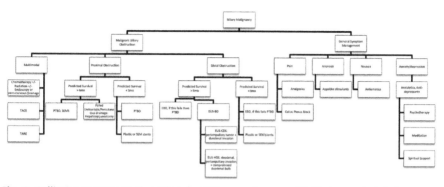

Fig. 1. Palliative treatment algorithm for biliary malignancy. TACE, transarterial chemoembolization; TARE, transarterial radioembolization.

indications, most commonly intrahepatic or distal biliary obstructions, and have a place in the diagnosis and in preoperative and palliative management.[25] Endoscopic biliary drainage (EBD) modalities via dilation of strictures or stent placement across tumors, or to relieve mass effect due to a tumor, have been used primarily for biliary decompression in patients with obstructive jaundice to relieve symptoms, such as severe itching or biliary sepsis, mainly from distally located tumors. Intrahepatic tumors more often are treated initially with percutaneous access of the biliary tree due to anatomic limitations that prevent successful endoscopic intervention. The timing and approach to managing MBO are critical. The following questions must be addressed clearly to avoid inappropriate use of endoluminal or percutaneous therapies: (1) Has a diagnosis of MBO been established? (2) Is the tumor resectable? and (3) Is the patient a surgical candidate? Failure to successfully answer these questions prior to intervention can have disastrous and life-limiting consequences. For example, if a tissue diagnosis of malignancy has not been obtained prior to endoluminal or percutaneous biliary intervention, obtaining a satisfactory biopsy can be difficult/impossible, particularly if a stent has been placed. Without biopsy confirmation of malignancy, cancer-directed therapies, if otherwise indicated, may not be offered. The accuracy of diagnostic imaging also can be impacted negatively by the placement of a stent or other biliary drainage (BD) procedure. For those patients who may be considered for surgical resection in the future, perioperative complications, in particular infectious complications, are increased in patients who have undergone preoperative biliary decompression.[25–27]

Stents commonly are used for unresectable tumors. In patients with unresectable disease, EBD with stent placement has shown to be less morbid than surgical intervention while providing similar relief of symptoms and survival. The primary outcomes measured in the setting of unresectable disease are survival and stent patency rather than actual palliative outcomes, such as symptomatic relief or quality of life. Consequently, the optimal endoscopic and/or endoluminal approach to palliation of MBO largely is unstudied.

The most common types of stents utilized in patients with MBO are plastic and self-expanding metal stents (SEMSs). Drug-eluting SEMSs are coated most commonly with chemotherapeutic agents, such as paclitaxel, gemcitabine, or sorafenib.[28,29] SEMSs are recommended for patients with predicted survival of greater than 3 months and Bismuth types II–IV hilar cholangiocarcinoma. Plastic stents typically are recommended as temporary drainage option for cholangitis, in cases of undetermined treatment plan, or when predicted survival is less than 3 months.[30] Published data support use of SEMSs over plastic stents due higher clinical success rates (77%), higher long-term patency rates (median 5.4 months), and reduced need for secondary procedures. Park and colleagues[31] reviewed the efficacy of various stents for palliation of MBO and reported that SEMss (covered and uncovered) were superior to plastic ones in terms of recurrent biliary obstruction. Due to the short median survival associated MBO in patients with unresectable disease, in many cases, SEMSs may provide lifetime patency and reduction of future endoscopic interventions.[32–34] Covered SEMSs have been shown to have increased patency rates (up to 85.7% at 12 months) compared with uncovered SEMSs, likely due to decreased tumor ingrowth across the interstices and the margins of the stent. Moole and colleagues[35] compared covered and uncovered stents and did not find any differences in survival, overall adverse events, or patency rates between these 2 types of stents. Some investigators argue that the benefits of covered SEMSs do not outweigh their increased costs.

A growing body of literature also has sought to determine the optimal technique for stent placement for MBO. Transmural stenting refers to EUS-guided BD (EUS-BD) and is a lesser-known endoscopic treatment option for MBO. This intervention is not widely available due to limited access to the device utilized and the need for specialized training in EUS-BD specifically.[36] EUS-BD includes choledochoduodenostomy stent (CDS) and hepaticogastrostomy stent (HGS). EUS-CDS is considered for patients with distal biliary obstruction and periampullary tumor infiltration with distal duodenal invasion. EUS-HGS is considered for patients with distal biliary obstruction and duodenal bulb invasion (ie, gastric outlet obstruction), periampullary duodenal invasion with compromised duodenal bulb, or surgically altered anatomy.[36] EUS-CDS and EUS-HGS utilize a lumen apposing metallic stent (LAMS) for drainage. Two recent systematic reviews and meta-analyses comparing LAMSs to SEMSs reported comparable rates of technical feasibility (in excess of 90%), complications (17.1% vs 18.3%, respectively), and reintervention (10.9% vs 13.9%, respectively).[37,38] Within the EUS-BD groups, there was no difference in stent patency rate between EUS-CDS and HGS.[36] Additionally, multiple reviews comparing EUS-BD versus ERCP-BD for the management of MBO have found equivalent efficacy of these 2 procedures, with some reviews reporting lower complications in the EUS-BD group (eg, post-ERCP pancreatitis and stent dysfunction) and shorter hospital stay (4 d vs 5 d).[39–44] Because EUS-guided procedures require creation of a temporary fistula, however, risk of bile leak is of major concern despite an approximately 5% complication rate.[45]

Stent occlusion is a significant issue in patients with MBO managed with stent placement and is important particularly in the palliative setting because repeat interventions associated with stent can have an adverse impact on quality of life, particularly for patients with limited life expectancy. As a result, various investigators have sought to identify techniques that can improve stent patency. Some investigators have reported a potential role for drug-eluting SEMSs to prevent direct tumor ingrowth and thereby increase patency rate.[33,46] In contrast, a recent review by Mohan and colleagues[47] found comparable overall survival and stent patency as well as complications between drug-eluting and covered metal stents.

Zhu and colleagues[48] reported on a multicenter trial of irradiation stents (I^{125}) versus conventional metal stents for MBO. Compared with SEMSs, irradiation stents have lower rates of occlusions (9% vs 15%, respectively, at 90 days; 16% vs 27%, respectively, at 180 days; and 21% vs 33%, respectively, at 360 days). Survival in patients treated with irradiation stents was longer: median survival was 202 days versus 140 days compared with SEMs.[48] Intraluminal brachytherapy and biliary stenting were compared with stenting alone by Xu and colleagues[49] in a systematic review and meta-analysis of 12 studies representing 641 patients. They found that the combination of brachytherapy and stenting was superior to stenting alone in terms of stent occlusion and mean survival with comparable complications and efficacy of normalization of liver function studies. The combination of intraductal radiofrequency ablation (RFA) plus stenting in MBO caused by cholangiocarcinoma recently was reviewed by Cha and colleagues[50] They found that overall survival was improved with RFA with stent insertion versus stenting alone. No difference in duration of stent patency was found between the 2 groups. Similar to the findings combining intraductal RFA plus stenting, the combination of high intensity focused ultrasound with stenting is associated with improved stent patency and overall survival in patients with MBO.[51] The current literature largely is based on pooled analyses of several studies, and key issues, such as the learning curve required to successfully administer these advanced techniques as well as how they should be incorporated treatment algorithms, are lacking.

Due to the issues related to stenting for MBO, some investigators have advocated for ablative procedures for biliary malignancies, primarily cholangiocarcinoma, prestent or poststent placement. For example, Laquiµre and colleagues[52] reported on a small series of patients with unresectable extrahepatic cholangiocarcinoma treated with endoscopic biliary RFA. The reported that this procedure had an acceptable safety profile with no adverse events or biliary fistula. Yang and colleagues[28] recently reported on 75 patients with unresectable extrahepatic cholangiocarcinoma treated with endoscopic RFA either with or without a novel 5-fluorouracil compound. They found a median overall survival of 16 months in the RFA plus chemotherapy group compared with 11 months in the RFA-alone group ($P<.001$). Karnofsky performance scale scores also were significantly higher in the combined treatment group at 9 months and 12 months, postoperatively. Recent reviews have confirmed the findings of these studies, showing improved stent patency and overall survival in this particularly challenging patient population, and note that the ideal treatment approach remains unclear owing to the novelty of these techniques and lack of widespread availability of the equipment and expertise required.[29,30]

SURGICAL VERSUS ENDOLUMINAL OR PERCUTANEOUS INTERVENTIONS

The choice of surgical versus endoluminal or percutaneous intervention for MBO is dependent on several factors, including morbidity and mortality of the procedure and length of hospitalization. The risks of palliative procedures are well known and have a significant impact, particularly in patients with limited life expectancy. Additionally, the time required to recover from an intervention also can have a negative impact on patient quality of life. Surgical bypass has a lower rate of recurrent biliary obstruction compared with endoscopic stent placement: 3.1% versus 28.7%, respectively, with a risk ratio of 0.14 in 1 study.[53] A 2-fold increase in total number of hospital days from the index procedure until death has been reported in patients undergoing stenting compared with surgical bypass due to the need for repeat procedures, including stent replacement or ultimate need for percutaneous BD (PTBD). Despite the superiority of surgical bypass in terms of lower rate of recurrent biliary obstruction, overall survival and rates of major morbidity and mortality are comparable to stenting alone. Significant complications are associated, however, with these palliative surgical interventions and include gastrointestinal bleeding, wound infections, gastrointestinal obstruction, pulmonary embolism, and stroke. Up to 50% of patients treated for MBO eventually require an intervention for gastric outlet obstruction; therefore, some investigators advocate performing simultaneous enteric bypass during surgical biliary bypass.[53] Robust evidence comparing surgery versus PTBD is not available. Current recommendations are surgical bypass with concomitant gastric emptying procedure if life expectancy is at least 6 months. SEMS is recommended if life expectancy is less than 4 months. No appropriate/clear recommendation if expected survival is 4 months to 6 months.[53]

THE ROLE OF PALLIATIVE CARE

The choice of placing supportive and palliative care first is deliberate and responds to the often prognosis of both pancreatic adenocarcinoma and cholangiocarcinoma, the 2 primary causes of MBO. The definition of palliative care according to the World Health Organization is "an approach that improves the quality of life of patients and their families facing the problem associated with life-threatening illness, through the prevention and relief of suffering by means of early identification and impeccable assessment and treatment of pain and other problems, physical, psychosocial and spiritual.[54] Therefore, it is expected that a multidisciplinary approach to patient-centered care is more likely to deliver the necessary holistic palliative care that these patients and families need.

In both eras of MBO management, the need for palliative care has been apparent. In the first era, curative intent rarely was an option; therefore, optimal methods to prepare patients and family for an inevitable death had to be initiated at the time of the diagnosis of incurability. Choices were limited, guided only by the aggressivity of the condition. In the second era, medical and technological advancement supported patients, their families, and the medical team and created a bridge to safer and less morbid means of MBO management. Additionally, advances in imaging and surgical techniques and perioperative care improved surgeons' ability to select patients for surgical intervention, both palliative and those with curative intent. A growing body of literature characterizes the benefits of palliative care in patients with advanced malignancies, in general, and in MBO, specifically.[55–58] In addition to the benefits of palliative care for symptom management, the importance of clear communication and prognostic awareness is paramount. A recent review by Laryionava and Winkler[59] found that eliciting patient preferences enabled advance care planning, avoided overtreatment at end of life, and helped ensure that patients received goal-concordant care. Particularly in the setting of the aggressive malignancies associated with MBO, understanding patient preferences for balancing the trade-off between quantity of life and quality of life is crucial.[60] Additionally, as choices become nonbinary: life, death, or survival with the disease, the central role of patient-centered decision-making is key and the challenge for providers is to resist portraying treatment options in these binary terms. This mode of thinking—la pensée unique—is a 1980 derivative of the economic thinking, "there is no alternative," that has affected not only oncology but also other modalities of aggressive care, especially critical care.[61] Coincident with the medical and technological advances seen between the 2 eras of MBO management has been a shift from the well-intentioned, if paternalistic, approach to medical decision making toward shared decision-making models. The essence of the trust between surgeons and patients is the disclosure of attainable goals, allowing for an informed decision. The discussion about attainable goals can be mediated through the utilization of scenarios, best case/worst case, as illustrated in Kruser and colleagues,[62] to assist in the definition of choices. Although autonomy is elevated as a primary ethical value in bioethics in the United States, choices of nonaggressive care often are questioned and challenged by medical teams, revealing cultural differences between patients and physicians.[63,64] It also is during this second era that the role of palliative care in cancer care has been recognized.[55] Despite that most major oncology professional societies and cancer care guidelines call for the integration of palliative care with routine cancer care, an integrated model of care still is far distant in all but the largest cancer centers.[65,66] Beesley and colleagues[67] used the term, *tsunami*, to describe unmet supportive care needs in patients with pancreatic and ampullary cancers. They found that 96% of those survey reported having some palliative care needs. Only 59% of patients with unresectable disease, however, accessed palliative care services compared with 27% for those with resectable tumors.

SUMMARY

MBO is an ominous sign and warrants prompt evaluation and management. The options for management depend on the location of the obstruction and on the tumor histology. Unfortunately, in a majority of cases, MBO portends poor prognosis. Technical considerations regarding the optimal management for biliary decompression tend to dominate the initial treatment decision making. These considerations must not be prioritized, however, to the exclusion of other significant needs of the patient and their family for aggressive symptom management (beyond addressing jaundice) and early initiation of goals of care discussions. The surgeon must be prepared to provide the full spectrum of palliative treatment required in these cases: surgical biliary and/or enteric bypass, referral for endoscopic or percutaneous biliary interventions, multidisciplinary coordinated care with medical and radiation oncology, and medical management for the symptoms seen most commonly, including tumor-related pain, nausea and vomiting, and fatigue.[68,69]

There is little doubt that advances in procedural interventions and systemic therapies will continue to improve for patients with MBO, just as seen between the first and second eras. These advances will come through properly designed studies, ideally that include a representative sample of those affected by these tumors. The need for holistic patient care, from the time of diagnosis to end of life, is essential. Those providers charged with caring for patients with MBO must remain vigilant against the temptation to measure that which is easy to measure (eg, bilirubin levels, overall survival, and progression-free survival) while minimizing the outcomes most important to the patient; it cannot be assumed that these are the same or equal. Early integration of palliative care, either through utilization of dedicated departments or, more importantly, by institutional initiative to develop a multidisciplinary primary palliative care, offers one of the surest ways to ensure that patient care stays patient focused.

DISCLOSURE

The authors have nothing to disclose.

REFERENCES

1. Gawande A. Being mortal:medicine and what matters in the end. New York: Metropolitan Books, Henry Holt and Company; 2014.

2. Sulik G. What cancer survivorship means. AMA J Ethics 2013;15(8):697–703.

3. McNamara MG, de Liguori Carino N, Kapacee ZA, et al. Outcomes in older patients with biliary tract cancer. Eur J Surg Oncol 2021;47:569–75.

4. Moffat GT, Epstein AS, O'Reilly EM. Pancreatic cancer—A disease in need: optimizing and integrating supportive care. Cancer 2019;125(22):3927–35.

5. Banales JM, Marin JJG, Lamarca A, et al. Cholangiocarcinoma 2020: the next horizon in mechanisms and management. Nat Rev Gastroenterol Hepatol 2020; 17(9):557–88.

6. Taylor A, Stapley S, Hamilton W. Jaundice in primary care: a cohort study of adults aged >45 years using electronic medical records. Fam Pract 2012; 29(4):416–20.

7. Fernandez Y, Viesca M, Arvanitakis M. Early diagnosis and management of malignant distal biliary obstruction: a review on current recommendations and guidelines. Clin Exp Gastroenterol 2019;12:415–32.

8. Siegel RL, Miller KD, Jemal A. Cancer statistics, 2020. CA Cancer J Clin 2020; 70(1):7–30.

9. Survival rates for pancreatic cancer. Available at: https://www.cancer.org/cancer/ pancreatic-cancer/detection-diagnosis-staging/survival-rates.html. Accessed September 29, 2020.

10. Survival rates for bile duct cancer. Available at: https://www.cancer.org/cancer/ bile-duct-cancer/detection-diagnosis-staging/survival-by-stage.html. Accessed September 29, 2020.

11. Holly EA, Chaliha I, Bracci PM, et al. Signs and symptoms of pancreatic cancer: a population-based case-control study in the San Francisco Bay area. Clin Gastroenterol Hepatol 2004;2(6):510–7.

12. Hart PA, Kamada P, Rabe KG, et al. Weight loss precedes cancer-specific symptoms in pancreatic cancer-associated diabetes mellitus. Pancreas 2011;40(5): 768–72.

13. Olson SH, Xu Y, Herzog K, et al. Weight loss, diabetes, fatigue, and depression preceding pancreatic cancer. Pancreas 2016;45(7):986–91.

14. Nehls O, Gregor M, Klump B. Serum and bile markers for cholangiocarcinoma. Semin Liver Dis 2004;24(2):139–54.

15. Marrelli D, Caruso S, Pedrazzani C, et al. CA19-9 serum levels in obstructive jaundice: clinical value in benign and malignant conditions. Am J Surg 2009;198(3): 333–9.

16. Goonetilleke KS, Siriwardena AK. Systematic review of carbohydrate antigen (CA 19-9) as a biochemical marker in the diagnosis of pancreatic cancer. Eur J Surg Oncol 2007;33(3):266–70.

17. Hasan S, Jacob R, Manne U, et al. Advances in pancreatic cancer biomarkers. Oncol Rev 2019;13(1):410.

18. Toft J, Hadden WJ, Laurence JM, et al. Imaging modalities in the diagnosis of pancreatic adenocarcinoma: a systematic review and meta-analysis of sensitivity, specificity and diagnostic accuracy. Eur J Radiol 2017;92:17–23.

19. Turner BG, Cizginer S, Agarwal D, et al. Diagnosis of pancreatic neoplasia with EUS and FNA: a report of accuracy. Gastrointest Endosc 2010;71(1):91–8.

20. Mallery JS, Centeno BA, Hahn PF, et al. Pancreatic tissue sampling guided by EUS, CT/US, and surgery: a comparison of sensitivity and specificity. Gastrointest Endosc 2002;56(2):218–24.

21. Maingot R. Techniques in British surgery. WB Saunders; 1950.

22. Cattell R, Warren K. Surgery of the pancreas. WB Saunders; 1954.

23. Saldinger P, Jarnagin W, Blumgart L. Hilar Cholangiocarcinoma. In: Hepatobiliary cancer. Hamilton, Canada: BC Decker; 2001. p. 193–209.

24. Harrington DP, Barth KH, Maddrey WC, et al. Percutaneously placed biliary stents in the management of malignant biliary obstruction. Dig Dis Sci 1979;24(11): 849–57.

25. Boulay BR, Birg A. Malignant biliary obstruction: From palliation to treatment. World J Gastrointest Oncol 2016;8(6):498.
26. Celotti A, Solaini L, Montori G, et al. Preoperative biliary drainage in hilar cholangiocarcinoma: Systematic review and meta-analysis. Eur J Surg Oncol 2017; 43(9):1628–35.
27. Shah T. Drug-eluting stents in malignant biliary obstruction: where do we stand? Dig Dis Sci 2013;58(3):610–2.
28. Yang JM, Wang JM, Zhou HM, et al. Endoscopic radiofrequency ablation plus a novel oral 5-fluorouracil compound versus radiofrequency ablation alone for unresectable extrahepatic cholangiocarcinoma. Gastrointest Endosc 2020;92(6): 1204–12.
29. Buerlein RCD, Wang AY. Endoscopic retrograde cholangiopancreatography-guided ablation for cholangiocarcinoma. Gastrointest Endosc Clin N Am 2019; 29(2):351–67.
30. Nabi Z, Reddy DN. Intraductal therapies. In: Ercp. Chichester, UK: John Wiley & Sons, Ltd; 2020. p. 149–63.
31. Park CH, Park SW, Jung JH, et al. Comparative efficacy of various stents for palliation in patients with malignant extrahepatic biliary obstruction: a systematic review and network meta-Analysis. J Pers Med 2021;11(2):86.
32. Fukasawa M, Takano S, Shindo H, et al. Endoscopic biliary stenting for unresectable malignant hilar obstruction. Clin J Gastroenterol 2017;10(6):485–90.
33. Lorenz J. Management of Malignant biliary obstruction. Semin Interv Radiol 2016; 33(04):259–67.
34. Tang Z, Yang Y, Meng W, et al. Best option for preoperative biliary drainage in Klatskin tumor: a systematic review and meta-analysis. Medicine (Baltimore) 2017;96(43):e8372.
35. Moole H, Bechtold ML, Cashman M, et al. Covered versus uncovered self-expandable metal stents for malignant biliary strictures: a meta-analysis and systematic review. Indian J Gastroenterol 2016;35(5):323–30.
36. Paik WH, Lee TH, Park DH, et al. EUS-guided biliary drainage versus ERCP for the primary palliation of malignant biliary obstruction: a multicenter randomized clinical trial. Am J Gastroenterol 2018;113(7):987–97.
37. Amato A, Sinagra E, Celsa C, et al. Efficacy and safety of lumen apposing metal stents or self-expandable metal stents for endoscopic ultrasound-guided choledocho-duodenostomy: a systematic review and meta-analysis. Endoscopy 2020. Epub ahead of print.
38. Krishnamoorthi R, Dasari CS, Thoguluva Chandrasekar V, et al. Effectiveness and safety of EUS-guided choledochoduodenostomy using lumen-apposing metal stents (LAMS): a systematic review and meta-analysis. Surg Endosc 2020; 34(7):2866–77.
39. Lou X, Yu D, Li J, et al. Efficacy of endoscopic ultrasound-guided and endoscopic retrograde cholangiopancreatography-guided biliary drainage for malignant biliary obstruction: a systematic review and meta-analysis. Minerva Med 2019;110(6):564–74.
40. Han SY, Kim S-O, So H, et al. EUS-guided biliary drainage versus ERCP for first-line palliation of malignant distal biliary obstruction: a systematic review and meta-analysis. Sci Rep 2019;9(1):16551.
41. Miller CS, Barkun AN, Martel M, et al. Endoscopic ultrasound-guided biliary drainage for distal malignant obstruction: a systematic review and meta-analysis of randomized trials. Endosc Int Open 2019;7(11):E1563–73.

42. Jin Z, Wei Y, Lin H, et al. Endoscopic ultrasound-guided versus endoscopic retrograde cholangiopancreatography-guided biliary drainage for primary treatment of distal malignant biliary obstruction: a systematic review and meta-analysis. Dig Endosc 2020;32(1):16–26.

43. Logiudice FP, Bernardo WM, Galetti F, et al. Endoscopic ultrasound-guided vs endoscopic retrograde cholangiopancreatography biliary drainage for obstructed distal malignant biliary strictures: a systematic review and meta-analysis. World J Gastrointest Endosc 2019;11(4):281–91.

44. Bishay K, Boyne D, Yaghoobi M, et al. Endoscopic ultrasound-guided transmural approach versus ERCP-guided transpapillary approach for primary decompression of malignant biliary obstruction: a meta-analysis. Endoscopy 2019;51(10):950–60.

45. Bertani H, Frazzoni M, Mangiafico S, et al. Cholangiocarcinoma and malignant bile duct obstruction: a review of last decades advances in therapeutic endoscopy. World J Gastrointest Endosc 2015;7(6):582–92.

46. Shatzel J, Kim J, Sampath K, et al. Drug eluting biliary stents to decrease stent failure rates: A review of the literature. World J Gastrointest Endosc 2016;8(2):77–85.

47. Mohan BP, Canakis A, Khan SR, et al. Drug eluting versus covered metal stents in malignant biliary strictures-Is there a clinical benefit?: a systematic review and meta-analysis. J Clin Gastroenterol 2021;55(3):271–7.

48. Zhu H-D, Guo J-H, Huang M, et al. Irradiation stents vs. conventional metal stents for unresectable malignant biliary obstruction: a multicenter trial. J Hepatol 2018;68(5):970–7.

49. Xu X, Li J, Wu J, et al. A systematic review and meta-analysis of intraluminal brachytherapy versus stent alone in the treatment of malignant obstructive jaundice. Cardiovasc Intervent Radiol 2018;41(2):206–17.

50. Cha BH, Jang M-J, Lee SH. Survival benefit of intraductal radiofrequency ablation for malignant biliary obstruction: a systematic review with metanalysis. Clin Endosc 2021;54(1):100–6.

51. Cai P-F, Gu H, Zhu L-J, et al. Stent insertion with high-intensity focused ultrasound ablation for malignant biliary obstruction: a protocol of systematic review and meta-analysis. Medicine (Baltimore) 2021;100(3):e23922.

52. Laquière A, Boustière C, Leblanc S, et al. Safety and feasibility of endoscopic biliary radiofrequency ablation treatment of extrahepatic cholangiocarcinoma. Surg Endosc 2016;30(3):1242–8.

53. Glazer ES, Hornbrook MC, Krouse RS. A meta-analysis of randomized trials: immediate stent placement vs. surgical bypass in the palliative management of malignant biliary obstruction. J Pain Symptom Manage 2014;47(2):307–14.

54. WHO. WHO Definition of Palliative Care. WHO. Available at: https://www.who.int/cancer/palliative/definition/en/. Accessed September 5, 2020.

55. Statement of Principles of Palliative Care. American College of Surgeons. Available at: https://www.facs.org/about-acs/statements/50-palliative-care. Accessed September 5, 2020.

56. Bakitas M, Lyons KD, Hegel MT, et al. Effects of a palliative care intervention on clinical outcomes in patients with advanced cancer: the Project ENABLE II randomized controlled trial. JAMA 2009;302(7):741–9.

57. Nakakura EK, Warren RS. Palliative care for patients with advanced pancreatic and biliary cancers. Surg Oncol 2007;16(4):293–7.

58. Greer JA, Pirl WF, Jackson VA, et al. Effect of early palliative care on chemotherapy use and end-of-life care in patients with metastatic non-small-cell lung cancer. J Clin Oncol 2012;30(4):394–400.
59. Laryionava K, Winkler EC. Patients' preferences in non-curable cancer disease. Oncol Res Treat 2019;42(1–2):31–4.
60. Shrestha A, Martin C, Burton M, et al. Quality of life versus length of life considerations in cancer patients: a systematic literature review. Psychooncology 2019; 28(7):1367–80.
61. Bacqué M-F. Contre la pensée unique. Psycho-Oncol. 2012;6(2):130–1.
62. Kruser JM, Taylor LJ, Campbell TC, et al. "Best Case/Worst Case": Training surgeons to use a novel communication tool for high-risk acute surgical problems. J Pain Symptom Manage 2017;53(4):711–9.
63. Woo JA, Stern TA, Maytal G. Clinical challenges to the delivery of end-of-life care: (Rounds in the General Hospital). Prim Care Companion J Clin Psychiatry 2006; 08(06):367–72.
64. Manassis K. The effects of cultural differences on the physician-patient relationship. Can Fam Physician 1986;32:5.
65. Ferrell BR, Temel JS, Temin S, et al. Integration of palliative care into standard oncology care: American Society of Clinical Oncology Clinical Practice Guideline Update. J Clin Oncol 2017;35(1):96–112.
66. Hui D, Bruera E. Models of integration of oncology and palliative care. Ann Palliat Med 2015;4(3):89–98.
67. Beesley VL, Janda M, Goldstein D, et al. A tsunami of unmet needs: pancreatic and ampullary cancer patients' supportive care needs and use of community and allied health services. Psychooncology 2016;25(2):150–7.
68. Lillemoe KD, Pitt HA. Palliation. Surgical and otherwise. Cancer 1996;78(3 Suppl):605–14.
69. Conrad C, Lillemoe KD. Surgical palliation of pancreatic cancer. Cancer J 2012; 18(6):577–83.

Artificial Nutrition in Patients with Advanced Malignancy

Ramses Saavedra, MD[a], Bridget N. Fahy, MD[a,b],*

KEYWORDS

• Artificial nutrition • Cancer • Palliative care • Patient selection

KEY POINTS

• Artificial nutrition usage is common in advanced cancer and palliative patients with malnutrition.
• Technical, patient, and oncologic factors all affect the decision to use artificial nutrition.
• Patient selection should include performance status and nutritional status evaluations and is critical to successful use of artificial nutrition.
• Shared decision-making is necessary for consent, given the complexity of these patients and possible complications associated with artificial nutrition.

INTRODUCTION

Cancer is a progressive disease that leads to an inflammatory state. Anorexia, weight loss, and, in late stages, cachexia, are common clinical findings. Malnutrition commonly affects patients with cancer, with 30% to 90% of patients experiencing malnutrition during their disease course.[1,2] This variation stems in part from the type of cancer. For example, 31% of patients with hematologic cancers will experience weight loss compared with up to 87% in those with gastric cancer.[3] Severe malnutrition in patients with advanced cancer can reflect this inflammatory state or can be a consequence of complications of the underlying malignancy. In response to tumor burden, the body has a mass release of catabolic hormones and proinflammatory cytokines that directly contribute to the anorexia/cachexia syndrome seen in cancer through their effects on metabolism.[4] Lean mass is reduced, as skeleton proteolysis is activated by this proinflammatory state.[1] Fat loss may be the result of direct tumor production of lipid mobilizing factor.[5] Mechanical effects of the tumor can lead to malnutrition by occluding the oropharynx and gastrointestinal tract causing dysphagia

[a] Department of Surgery, University of New Mexico, 1 University of New Mexico, MSC 07-4025, Albuquerque, NM 87131, USA; [b] Division of Palliative Medicine, University of New Mexico, Albuquerque, NM, USA
* Corresponding author. Department of Surgery, University of New Mexico, 1 University of New Mexico, MSC 07-4025, Albuquerque, NM 87131.
E-mail address: bfahy@salud.unm.edu

Surg Oncol Clin N Am 30 (2021) 505–518
https://doi.org/10.1016/j.soc.2021.02.005
surgonc.theclinics.com

or malignant bowel obstruction. In addition, chemotherapy-induced nausea and emesis can also adversely affect nutritional status. Chemotherapy can act directly on neuroreceptors of the brain through central and peripheral pathways, causing both delayed and acute chemotherapy-induced emesis, respectively.[6] Sensation of taste and smell are also altered for many undergoing chemotherapy, contributing further to eating difficulties and subsequent malnutrition.[7]

With the profound effects malnutrition and associated weight loss have on patients with cancer, clinicians regularly encounter challenges of preventing and managing this issue. Introduction of artificial nutrition (AN) in patients with advanced cancer is considered for a variety of indications and with varying goals. In some cases, it is used as a means of supporting patients while they receive cancer-directed therapy. In other cases, it is needed to compensate for adverse effects directly from the tumor or its treatment. For patients with very advanced cancers, it can be provided for palliative indications. Regardless of the indication or goal of AN, it is important to note that *AN is a medical therapy* that uses artificial means of delivery to assist the patient in achieving adequate nutrition. AN is different from eating, as it is independent of the patient's ability to tolerate oral intake. Furthermore, nutrition is not the same as food. Food often carries with it a significant cultural, even spiritual significance and is more intimately intertwined with perceptions of well-being and care for many people. In addition, as any medical therapy, AN is associated with both risks and benefits. The decision to initiate AN in patients with advanced cancer should consider patient factors, technical aspects of type and method of delivering AN, and oncologic considerations.

PATIENT FACTORS

Selecting patients most likely to benefit from AN requires an assessment of their physical fitness for therapy as well as a clear understanding of how AN fits into their overall goals of care. Careful assessment of performance status can help identify patients more likely to benefit from AN, as those patients who require more assistance in their daily activities will tend to have shorter life expectancy and therefore less likely to benefit from AN. Performance status is critical in selecting patients for any therapy and may be a potent predictor of who will benefit from therapy. Many tools exist to measure performance status. The Karnofsky Performance Status (KPS) been shown to correlate, if not predict, oncologic outcomes, including survival.[8] Chermesh and colleagues[9] found that patients with malignant bowel obstruction and higher KPS have improved survival compared with those with lower performance status.

Nutritional screening at the initial assessment for AN may help predict who will benefit from therapy. **Table 1** shows the components of multiple screening tools that have all been shown to be valid, with the Malnutrition Screening Tool (MST) being the most reliable.[10] Screening tools can help identify which patients are suffering from weight loss and are at risk for developing cachexia as well as those who already meet criteria for cachexia. The severity of cancer cachexia can be labeled as precachexia, cachexia, and refractory cachexia using parameters of weight loss, body mass index (BMI), energy expenditure, and presence of sarcopenia.[11] Refractory cachexia is associated with low performance scores and life expectancy of less than 3 months.[11]

Determining lean body mass can also be helpful in assessing nutritional status; low muscle mass is associated with lower quality of life and shorter survival.[16] The goal of AN is, in part, to prevent lean body mass loss for this reason. Early use of AN may help improve body composition as well as serum prealbumin levels.[17] Using bioimpedance vector analysis,[18] body cell mass can be determined and has been suggested as

	Weight Loss	Nutritional Intake	BMI	Severity of Disease	Acute Disease	Functional Status	Arm Circumference
NRS-2002[12]	X	X	x	x	x		
MNA-SF[13]	X	X	x		x	x	
MST[14]	X	X					
MUST[15]	X		x		x		X

Table 1
Nutritional screening tool components

Abbreviations: BMI, body mass index; MNA-SF, Mini-Nutritional Assessment—Short Form; MST, malnutrition screening tool; MUST, malnutrition universal screening tool; NRS-2002, nutritional risk screening-2002.

another option for determining nutrition status when other clinical parameters are not reliable.[19]

Patients with cancer often have comorbidities, and so it is valuable to evaluate the indications and outcomes of AN in other populations. One group where enteric feeding is commonly discussed is those with advanced dementia. The perceived nutritional and palliative benefits of tube feedings lead to this intervention commonly being performed. A Cochrane review in 2009 showed that in patients with advanced dementia, there was no benefit in terms of mortality and no nutritional benefit.[20] The current data strongly suggest that there is little to no benefit for this patient population despite the large number of patients with advanced dementia who receive AN in the form of tube feedings.[20] Similarly, Teno and colleagues conducted a large prospective study evaluating patients with dementia and the potential variable effects depending on duration of feeding difficulty. No survival benefit was found with early initiation of tube feedings after eating difficulties began, suggesting the disease process itself will lead the death regardless of timing of AN.[21] The lessons learned from use of AN in patients with advanced dementia should be considered when considering AN in patients with advanced cancer who also have life-limiting comorbidities.

The beliefs and preferences of the patient and their families must also be considered when making recommendations regarding AN. Establishing their goals and values is essential to ensure appropriate use of this therapy, as patient autonomy needs to be respected. Starting, withholding, and withdrawing AN are all appropriate aspects of patient care but present challenging decision points to those involved. For example, some Asian cultures hold that it is a child's obligation to prevent death from hunger in their parents[22]; this leads to feeding tubes being placed despite a patient's wishes and retrospective acknowledgments from caregivers that many patients did not enjoy improved quality of life due to provision of AN.[22] Religious beliefs can also affect patient decision-making regarding AN. Those with no religious affiliation are more likely to decline aggressive medical management with a terminal diagnosis, whereas fundamentalist Catholic or Protestant patients often desire treatments they perceive as life-prolonging.[23] The distinction between withholding and withdrawing therapies is crucial, particularly for patients from certain faith traditions who may be concerned that withholding or withdrawing certain therapies, such as AN, is tantamount with suicide. Many Christian theologians argue that foregoing intervention is not a form of suicide when the potential benefit is outweighed by the burden of disease.[24] In addition, Buddhist views on the dying process are such that life-sustaining interventions are not always encouraged.[25] According to Chakraborty and colleagues,[23] it is not uncommon for Buddhists to refuse AN or even other potential comfort measures such as opioid pain medications, as their preference is to decline life-prolonging treatment if the chances of survival are low and to avoid an altered mental status at the time of death. Such personal beliefs can lead patients or their caregivers to continue or discontinue interventions, including AN, at a point that may not be clear to their physicians. Potential conflicts around the initiation, withholding, or withdrawing of AN may be lessened through early discussions identifying patient beliefs and values around nutrition and review of advance directives where wishes regarding AN are documented.[26]

TECHNICAL FACTORS

AN can either be provided enterally or parenterally. Enteral nutrition remains the preferred route in surgical and nonsurgical patients, when possible, due to decreased infection rates and the maintenance of gut integrity compared with parenteral access.[27] Parenteral nutrition (PN) is a means of administering AN through the peripheral or central venous system and is required in patients with intestinal failure and malignant bowel obstruction.

European Society for Parenteral and Enteral Nutrition (ESPEN) guidelines recommend AN when malnutrition is present, the patient is unable to eat for 7 days or more, there is weight loss greater than 10% initial body weight regardless of time or weight loss greater than 5% over 3 months with BMI less than 20, or when inadequate caloric intake for 10 days is present.[1,28] However, these guidelines are not typically intended for palliative patients and must be weighed in light of the patient's oncologic and anatomic factors, including prior surgical interventions and associated altered anatomy and nutritional physiology. In patients with advanced malignancy, life expectancy is another key variable to bear in mind when considering the risks and benefits of obtaining enteral access for AN. If life expectancy is expected to exceed 2 to 3 months, AN in those unable to eat by mouth may be reasonable.[29] Once the dying phase is approached, the risk:benefit calculation can change dramatically, as the benefits will not likely be as profound and risks and burdens of this therapy are expected to increase.

Short-term enteral access can be achieved via a temporary nasogastric or nasojejunal tube. This tube is especially helpful in the critically ill or perioperative patients. Early feeding in the critically ill patient may help prevent infection, sepsis, and may reduce hospital length of stay.[30] Nasoenteric feeding tubes are favored in these settings due to their ability to be placed at the bedside and lack of need for advanced imaging or invasive intervention for placement. As with all interventions, however, there are risks associated with nasoenteric feeding tubes. Epistaxis can occur in 1.8% to 4.7% of patients due to the trauma of placement. Prolonged placement of the nasoenteric tube carries a risk of sinusitis.[31] Although these can be relatively minor complications, they can contribute to significant discomfort for the patient. By the nature of how they are placed, these tubes can be quite irritating for the patient, leading to increased need for topical and systemic analgesics. Tube clogging is another common issue due to the smaller caliber and longer lengths of nasoenteric tubes. Especially in agitated patients, accidental or intentional tube removal becomes a concern. In some cases, use of physical or chemical restraints increases to prevent unintentional removal of these tubes.[31]

The most concerning complications of nasoenteric tubes are the associated pulmonary complications, stemming from malposition and aspiration pneumonia. A malpositioned tube can be coiled in the pharynx or esophagus or placed in the trachea or bronchial tree. Even with proper placement, aspiration pneumonia can occur in 10%

to 40% of intensive care unit patients and is a significant contributor to mortality.[32] One method suggested to decrease rates of aspiration pneumonia is post–pyloric tube placement through medically assisted, fluoroscopic, or endoscopic techniques. A Cochrane review in 2015 found a 30% decrease in pneumonia without an increase in complications from post–pyloric feeding tube placement; however, placement did not improve mortality and can be technically challenging in some cases.[33]

Establishing enteral access often requires an invasive procedure performed by a surgeon, gastroenterologist, or interventional radiologist. Although often perceived as being a "minor procedure," placement of feeding tubes, by whatever means, has been shown to carry significant risk, particularly in patients with significant underlying disease, such as cancer. The American College of Surgeons (ACS) Surgical Risk Calculator is a useful tool for estimating complications following surgical procedures.[34] For example, a 65-year-old man with malnutrition and disseminated cancer undergoing a laparoscopic gastrostomy tube placement has a 14.6% risk of a postoperative complication and 6% risk of 30-day mortality. These high risks of perioperative morbidity and mortality highlight the need for careful preoperative informed consent. Complications from percutaneous endoscopic gastrostomy (PEG) placement are multiple and include a variety of issues from potentially minor (eg, ileus, superficial wound infections, leakage, pain, tube clogging) to major (eg, aspiration, peritonitis, hemorrhage, malpositioned tubes, bowel perforation). Mortality rates vary depending on the indication for placement with overall complications rates ranging from 8% to 30%.[35] Despite not interfering with the esophageal sphincters, aspiration rates with PEG tubes are the same as those with nasoenteric tubes.[36] In patients undergoing PEG tube placement for malignancy other than head and neck cancer, mortality rates over time are high compared with most all other indications (eg, stroke, trauma, neuromuscular disorders) by 4- to 10-fold over the course of 3 years.[37]

Table 2 provides a summary of several selected studies used to compare various enteric feeding access methods as well as their outcomes. Although these studies

Table 2
Comparison of morbidity and mortality of selected studies

Study	Population (N)	Technique Comparison	Minor Complications (%)	Major Complications (%)	30-Day Mortality (%)
Grant et al,[38] 2009	Head and neck cancer (2353)	PEG	19.5	7.4	2.2
		RIG	22.1	8.9	1.8
Wollman et al,[39] 1995	Various indications (5752)	PEG	5.9	9.4	14.6
		RIG	7.8	5.9	15.4
		Open	9	19.9	16.2
Mansoor et al,[40] 2014	Various cancers (260)	PEG	21	3.8	–
Mizrahi et al,[41] 2014	Various indications (71)	Open	4.3	6.5	4.3
		Lap G	12	0	0
Choi et al,[42] 2017	Gastroesophageal cancers (117)	Lap J	35.9	25.6	0.9
Haskins et al,[43] 2018	Various indications (412)	Lap J	–	7.5	4.1
		PEG-JET	–	31.5	13.7

Minor complications are Clavien-Dindo class I–II. Major complications are Clavien-Dindo class III–V.
Abbreviations: Lap G, laparoscopic gastrostomy; Lap J, laparoscopic jejunostomy; Open, open gastrostomy; PEG, percutaneous endoscopic gastrostomy; PEG-JET, percutaneous endoscopic gastrostomy with jejunal extension; RIG, radiographically inserted gastrostomy.

vary in their patient populations and study designs, the overall complication rates and mortality are high for those needing enteric access, regardless of technique.

PN is most often administered through a central venous catheter, which introduces the risk for procedural and catheter-related complications. With image-guidance, complication rates are approximately 7%, with more severe complications such as pneumothorax, arterial puncture, or line malpositioning, ranging from 1% to 4%.[44] Once a line is in place, infections and complications requiring hospitalization range from 6% to 21%.[45] Bozzetti and colleagues[46] reported that 15% of patients who received home PN developed a catheter-related infection. Daily access and use of nutritional supplementation is also associated with higher hazard ratios and increased risk of catheter removal when compared with nonnutritional use.[46] Catheter dysfunction is another common complication after placement. Catheter dysfunction occurs at rates of 0.83 per 1000 catheter days, compared with 0.26 and 0.19 per 1000 catheter days for catheter site and blood stream infections, respectively.[47] Thrombosis is the most common cause of catheter dysfunction, often occurring within 7 days of placement and can result in early termination of therapy in 43% of patients and need for removal, replacement, or even hospitalization.[47]

Metabolic derangements can occur with PN. Hyperglycemia, electrolyte abnormalities, hyperlipidemia, hypercapnia, refeeding syndrome, and other metabolic derangements can have dramatic impacts on patients' lives. End-organ damages such as renal insufficiency, gastrointestinal failure and atrophy, and liver injury can occur.[44] Abnormalities in liver function studies occur in 20% to 90% of patients, although these are often asymptomatic; prolonged parenteral therapy can result in fibrosis and cirrhosis and can take up to 5 years to manifest.[44] Despite its effects on long-term liver function, PN may help improve mental status in malnourished cirrhotic and encephalopathic patients and may reduce infections in the perioperative period.[48] In patients with underlying renal insufficiency, the metabolic and electrolyte derangements associated with renal replacement therapies must also be considered. In particular, nitrogen balance is vital, as protein wasting is an independent risk for morbidity and mortality.[49] Appropriate fluid balance needs to be maintained as well, as those with renal failure are prone to fluid derangements,[49] and this may lead to issues such as third spacing that may be challenging to correct with ongoing malnutrition. It is therefore important that if this is pursued as a therapeutic intervention for the patient, laboratory testing and close monitoring be implemented to ensure patient safety. The burden of this monitoring must be factored into the overall recommendation for initiating or continuing PN.

ONCOLOGIC FACTORS

In patients with advanced cancer, it is vital to consider tumor-related variables when considering the use of AN. Although there may be a subset of patients with advanced cancer that benefit from AN, the data regarding its benefit in different malignancies are limited. Therefore, it is most useful to consider the prognosis of the underlying malignancy. A trial by Oh and colleagues[50] randomized patients with terminal cancer with a life expectancy of less than 3 months to either receive fluid therapy or PN. Patients randomized to parenteral fluid alone had a median survival of 8 days versus 13 days in the PN group. The study was terminated early due to familial concerns with starvation,[50] highlighting the challenges associated with studying patients with advanced cancer, particularly at the end of life. In a recent review, Bozzetti[51] argued against the use of AN in patients whose life expectancy was believed to be determined by their tumor rather than starvation. The study by Oh and colleagues, however, demonstrates the difficulty associated with accurately distinguishing between these 2 possible causes of death in patients with advanced cancer.

One malignancy where AN can be beneficial is head and neck cancer. Poor nutritional status has been associated with worse prognosis in this patient population.[52] AN in the form of enteric feeding can improve patient outcomes when adequate oral intake is no longer possible during treatment or due to disease progression. The delivery method for AN, via nasoenteric tube or PEG tube, does not seem to affect overall outcomes for patients.[52] Major complication rates are no different for patients with head and neck cancer receiving a PEG compared with patients with mixed pathologies, both cancerous and noncancerous.[38] Patients with prophylactically placed PEG tubes, compared with placement of tubes after feeding difficulties arise, may also benefit from lower stricture rates, aspiration rates, hospitalizations, and less overall costs.[53]

The benefit of AN in patients receiving cancer-directed therapy is unclear. In a systematic review in 2001, the American Gastrointestinal Association evaluated the concomitant use of PN during chemotherapy and radiation therapy.[54] They concluded that there was likely no survival benefit, but there was an associated increased risk of complications, including infection and a possible lower tumor response rate.[54] These data led the investigators to recommend against the routine use of PN in patients receiving chemotherapy and radiation therapy.[54] In a 2018 prospective trial of 65 adult patients with malnutrition and solid tumors receiving anticancer therapy, home PN was associated with improved BMI, body composition by Bioimpedance Analysis, and improved performance by KPS over 90 days.[55] The applicability of these findings to other malnourished patients with cancer is unclear, given the likely selection bias toward patients who were deemed candidates for anticancer therapy.

OUTCOMES WITH ARTIFICIAL NUTRITION

The benefits of AN in patients with advanced or end-stage malignancies are controversial. Factors that influence the request for AN in this situation are often affected by emotional and psychosocial factors rather than the objective benefits of this medical therapy. For example, it is not uncommon for patients and/or their family members to request for PN due to concerns that the patient will "starve to death" if this therapy is not provided. In addition, there is no clear consensus among medical providers about when or if PN should be provided to patients with advanced malignancies, particularly those without further cancer-directed therapy options. Bozzetti argued that home PN in patients with incurable cancer may be "indispensable to guarantee even short-term survival" and may be more beneficial in patients with > 3-month life expectancy.[29] It is still unclear if there is a survival benefit or if this is providing true palliation of symptoms. Orrevall and colleagues,[56] in a series of interviews with patients and family undergoing home PN for greater than 2 weeks, found a sense of relief that nutritional needs were being met and an overall tendency toward a positive experience with home PN. Distinguishing symptoms commonly seen at the end of life, such as dry mouth, with thirst or hunger is critical because the optimal treatment of the former is oral hygiene care, not AN.[26]

Several retrospective studies have evaluated the outcomes following AN in patients with cancer. Keung and colleagues evaluated 189 patients with both hematologic and nonhematologic malignancies after PEG placement; greater than 40% had metastatic disease. They found that 22% were able to become independent from total PN and 24% were able to have their diets advanced. However, major complication rates were approximately 10% and in-hospital mortality was 19%.[57] Nearly 25% of patients opted to have their code status changed to do not resuscitate after PEG placement.[57]

With variable benefits for each patient, it is challenging to predict who will have a desirable outcome. A study by Richards and colleagues[58] found that the risk of major complications and mortality increases with American Society of Anesthesia (ASA) scores greater than 4, international normalized ratio greater than 1.5, elevated leukocytosis, and advance tumor stages, indicating that sicker patients are at higher risk of adverse outcomes.[58]

The impact of home PN on quality of life in palliative patients has been the focus of several studies. In one multicenter French study, 767 malnourished patients with cancer receiving PN were given a self-administered questionnaire Functional Assessment of Cancer Therapy—General (FACT-G)[59] to evaluate changes in quality of life before and after initiation of therapy. The investigators found a perceived positive impact of 78% after 28 days associated with improved weight as well as serum albumin.[60] The durability of these improvements beyond 28 days is unknown. Bozzetti and colleagues[61] studied 69 severely malnourished patients with advanced stage cancer and observed them from initiation of home PN until death. The median survival time was 4 months and quality of life, measured using the Rotterdam Symptom Checklist

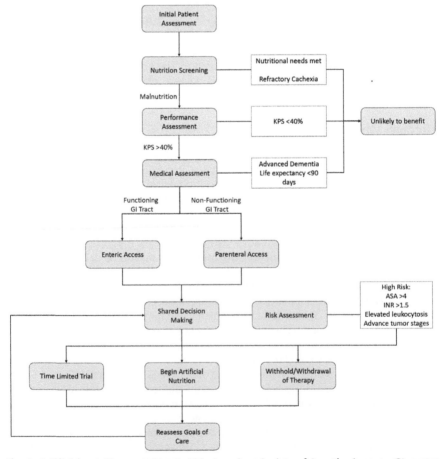

Fig. 1. Artificial nutrition assessment. ASA, American Society of Anesthesia score; GI, gastrointestinal; KPS, Karnofsky Performance Score.

questionnaire, remained stable until about 2 to 3 months before death.[61] Two meta-analyses that have examined changes in quality of life in patients with malignant bowel obstruction on home PN both suggested limited improvement, if any with home PN.[45,62]

Available data provide conflicting results on potential improved survival with AN. Naghibi and colleagues evaluated 12 studies looking at palliative patients with inoperable malignant bowel obstruction started on home PN. The pooled data of 244 patients found a mean survival of 116 days with a median of 83 days with 24% surviving at least 6 months.[62] A 2018 Cochrane review of survival in 721 patients in 13 separate studies with malignant bowel obstruction on home PN showed a median survival between 15 and 155 days. The investigators concluded that there was insufficient data to conclude there is a true survival benefit.[45] For both meta-analysis, there was a lack of appropriate comparative arms against those receiving home PN. In the absence of nutrition, it is suspected that these patients would likely die from starvation in 60 to 90 days at the longest estimates.[1,45,62,63] In summary, these data suggest that some minimum survival time is necessary for patients to see a benefit from PN. What is less clear is the exact amount of time needed and whether PN is providing a better quality of life as opposed to merely marginal improvement in survival.

More recent data from 2020 provide some clearer guidance about which patients may benefit from AN. In a large retrospective review of patients on home parenteral and enteral nutrition with advanced cancer, Ruggeri and colleagues found a survival rate of greater than 6 months in 73% of the patients. Their selection criteria included KPS of greater than or equal to 40%, life expectancy of 6 weeks or longer, inadequate caloric intake ± malnutrition, suitable psychophysical conditions (eg, no severe organ failure, pain controlled, appropriate hygiene, and able to understand and manage the home AN), and informed consent.[64] They reported no change in KPS after 1 month in 67%, increased performance status in 24%, and reduced performance status in 9%. The degree of cachexia before initiation of AN had a significant impact on changes in performance status. Patients with refractory cachexia did not show improvement in their KPS after 1 month compared with those with precachexia or cachexia. Complications were seen in 14% of patients on home enteral nutrition and 11% of patients on PN.

SUMMARY

AN can be a life-extending medical therapy. With AN, selecting the appropriate delivery method and patient is paramount. Families and patients should have as clear a picture as possible of who is likely to benefit and who will not. **Fig. 1** provides a recommended algorithm for assessment of AN. First, it must be ensured that the patient is indeed unable to meet adequate nutrition for a minimum of 10 days or unable to eat for 7 days.[1,63] Evaluation of a patient's performance status using a standardized performance status assessment tool such as KPS can help select for those more likely to benefit. Patients with KPS less than 40 will likely not benefit from AN and have a higher likelihood of complications. Similarly, early evaluation of nutritional status using tools such as the MST can help select for those that will benefit both in survival and in quality of life. Those with refractory cachexia are unlikely to experience an improvement in either quality of life or survival. Comorbidities need to be considered and those with advanced dementia, for example, should avoid use of AN. The personal and religious beliefs of the patient should also be considered to ensure that patient and family preferences are appreciated before initiating therapy as well as circumstances under which the therapy would be withheld or discontinued.

The enteric tract is the preferred route for AN, when possible. In the setting of a malignant bowel obstruction or intestinal failure, PN is required. Patients must be advised of both the procedural risks associated with AN access (eg, enteral tube or venous access) as well as the potential complications of AN itself. Tools such as the ACS risk calculator[34] can help determine a specific patient's risk for perioperative complication following placement of a feeding tube and help inform the consent process for both patients and surgeons. These same principles need to be used when consenting patients for PN. The discussion should include not just the immediate procedure complications, but the risks of sepsis and catheter-related thrombosis that can occur throughout the treatment.

Oncologic factors need to be considered during the selection process for AN. Although there seem to be clear benefits to AN in specific populations, such as those with head and neck cancers, the outcomes of AN in this group cannot be extrapolated to all other cancer populations. Patients with other cancers may benefit from AN but further studies are needed to better establish which patient groups are most likely to benefit. For those undergoing anticancer therapies, AN does not uniformly result in improved outcomes (eg, survival or increased performance status). Currently, there are no clear guidelines that patients receiving anticancer therapy will benefit from AN. The primary challenge in many of these situations is determining if patient survival is dictated by the underlying malignancy versus untreated malnutrition.

The consent process for AN is critical. Patient, technical, and oncologic factors must all be considered for appropriate and ethical use of this therapy. Before beginning AN, the goals of AN need to be specifically discussed, as this will differ from patient to patient. These can be reevaluated at appropriate time points to ensure goals of therapy are being met. It is vital to discuss the anticipated impact on survival, quality of life, and ability to receive additional cancer therapy in the context of the associated morbidity and mortality of AN access and treatment. There is a significant degree of uncertainty and risk associated with AN that makes informed consent challenging in this setting[65]; this is especially true when the goal of therapy is palliation and quality of life rather than life prolongation. A more thorough shared decision-making process is appropriate and necessary when accounting for the multiple options available to patients.[65] For some, it may be appropriate to offer a trial on AN through nasoenteric or parenteral access. The patient may decide that it is not in their best interest to continue with AN after a trial. It is important to remember that discontinuation of AN is both morally and ethically permissible when the therapy is no longer meeting a patient's goals and/or the burden of therapy is felt to outweigh the benefits.[66] Withholding AN in cases where it is unlikely to provide benefit, and may in fact prolong suffering in the dying phase, is also appropriate.[66] AN does play a role in palliative care of patients with advanced cancer. It ought to be the goal of clinicians not to be technicians in care of these patients but to guide them to the best option for their survival and comfort (see **Fig. 1**).

CLINICS CARE POINTS

- Before initiating AN in patients with advanced malignancy, the risks, benefits, and alternatives should be thoroughly considered, as would be performed before initiating any medical therapy.

- Patients should undergo nutritional screening before initiating AN, as those with refractory cachexia, low performance status, and limited life expectancy (typically <3 months) are unlikely to benefit from AN.

- Enteral nutrition is preferred over PN, when possible, due to the risks of catheter-related infections, metabolic derangements, and need for close laboratory monitoring associated with parenteral nutrition.

DISCLOSURE

The authors have nothing to disclose.

REFERENCES

1. Arends J, Bodoky G, Bozzetti F, et al. ESPEN guidelines on enteral nutrition: non-surgical oncology. Clin Nutr 2006;25(2):245–59.
2. Nitenberg G, Raynard B. Nutritional support of the cancer patient: issues and dilemmas. Crit Rev Oncol Hematol 2000;34(3):137–68.
3. Dewys WD, Begg C, Lavin PT, et al. Prognostic effect of weight loss prior to chemotherapy in cancer patients. Am J Med 1980;69(4):491–7.
4. Moldawer LL, Copeland EM 3rd. Proinflammatory cytokines, nutritional support, and the cachexia syndrome: interactions and therapeutic options. Cancer 1997;79(9):1828–39.
5. Khan S, Tisdale MJ. Catabolism of adipose tissue by a tumour-produced lipid-mobilising factor. Int J Cancer 1999;80(3):444–7.
6. Navari RM, Aapro M. Antiemetic prophylaxis for chemotherapy-induced nausea and vomiting. N Engl J Med 2016;374(14):1356–67.
7. Steinbach S, Hummel T, Böhner C, et al. Qualitative and quantitative assessment of taste and smell changes in patients undergoing chemotherapy for breast cancer or gynecologic malignancies. J Cin Oncol 2009;27(11):1899–905.
8. Viganó A, Bruera E, Jhangri GS, et al. Clinical survival predictors in patients with advanced cancer. Arch Intern Med 2000;160(6):861–8.
9. Chermesh I, Mashiach T, Amit A, et al. Home parenteral nutrition (HTPN) for incurable patients with cancer with gastrointestinal obstruction: do the benefits outweigh the risks? Med Oncol 2011;28(1):83–8.
10. Skipper A, Ferguson M, Thompson K, et al. Nutrition screening tools: an analysis of the evidence. JPEN J Parenter Enteral Nutr 2012;36(3):292–8.
11. Fearon K, Strasser F, Anker SD, et al. Definition and classification of cancer cachexia: an international consensus. Lancet Oncol 2011;12(5):489–95.
12. Kondrup J, Rasmussen HH, Hamberg O, et al, Ad Hoc ESPEN Working Group. Nutritional risk screening (NRS 2002): a new method based on an analysis of controlled clinical trials. Clin Nutr 2003;22(3):321–36.
13. Rubenstein LZ, Harker JO, Salvà A, et al. Screening for undernutrition in geriatric practice: developing the short-form mini-nutritional assessment (MNA-SF). J Gerontol A Biol Sci Med Sci 2001;56(6):M366–72.
14. Ferguson M, Capra S, Bauer J, et al. Development of a valid and reliable malnutrition screening tool for adult acute hospital patients. Nutrition 1999;15(6): 458–64.
15. Elia M. Screening for malnutrition: a multidisciplinary responsibility. Development and use of the Malnutrition Universal Screening Tool ('MUST') for adults. Redditch (England): BAPEN; 2003.
16. Prado CM, Purcell SA, Alish C, et al. Implications of low muscle mass across the continuum of care: a narrative review. Ann Med 2018;50(8):675–93.
17. Caccialanza R, Cereda E, Caraccia M, et al. Early 7-day supplemental parenteral nutrition improves body composition and muscle strength in hypophagic cancer patients at nutritional risk. Support Care Cancer 2019;27(7):2497–506.
18. Norman K, Stobäus N, Pirlich M, et al. Bioelectrical phase angle and impedance vector analysis–clinical relevance and applicability of impedance parameters. Clin Nutr 2012;31(6):854–61.

19. Caccialanza R, Pedrazzoli P, Cereda E, et al. Nutritional support in cancer patients: a position paper from the Italian Society of Medical Oncology (AIOM) and the Italian Society of Artificial Nutrition and Metabolism (SINPE). J Cancer 2016;7(2):131–5.

20. Sampson EL, Candy B, Jones L. Enteral tube feeding for older people with advanced dementia. Cochrane Database Syst Rev 2009;(2):CD007209.

21. Teno JM, Gozalo PL, Mitchell SL, et al. Does feeding tube insertion and its timing improve survival? J Am Geriatr Soc 2012;60(10):1918–21.

22. Somers E, Grey C, Satkoske V. Withholding versus withdrawing treatment: artificial nutrition and hydration as a model. Curr Opin Support Palliat Care 2016; 10(3):208–13.

23. Chakraborty R, El-Jawahri AR, Litzow MR, et al. A systematic review of religious beliefs about major end-of-life issues in the five major world religions. Palliat Support Care 2017;15(5):609–22.

24. O'Rourke KD. Artificial nutrition and hydration and the catholic tradition. The Terri Schiavo case had even members of Congress debating the issue. Health Prog 2007;88(3):50–4.

25. McCormick AJ. Buddhist ethics and end-of-life care decisions. J Soc Work End Life Palliat Care 2013;9(2–3):209–25.

26. Casarett D, Kapo J, Caplan A. Appropriate use of artificial nutrition and hydration — Fundamental principles and recommendations. N Engl J Med 2005;353(24): 2607–12.

27. Stroud M, Duncan H, Nightingale J, British Society of Gastroenterology. Guidelines for enteral feeding in adult hospital patients. Gut 2003;52:vii1–12.

28. Singer P, Blaser AR, Berger MM, et al. ESPEN guideline on clinical nutrition in the intensive care unit. Clin Nutr 2019;38(1):48–79.

29. Bozzetti F. Home total parenteral nutrition in incurable cancer patients: a therapy, a basic humane care or something in between? Clin Nutr 2003;22(2):109–11.

30. Marik PE, Zaloga GP. Early enteral nutrition in acutely ill patients: a systematic review. Crit Care Med 2001;29(12):2264–70.

31. Baskin WN. Acute complications associated with bedside placement of feeding tubes. Nutr Clin Pract 2006;21(1):40–55.

32. Ukleja A, Sanchez-Fermin P. Gastric versus post-pyloric feeding: relationship to tolerance, pneumonia risk, and successful delivery of enteral nutrition. Curr Gastroenterol Rep 2007;9(4):309–16.

33. Alkhawaja S, Martin C, Butler RJ, et al. Post-pyloric versus gastric tube feeding for preventing pneumonia and improving nutritional outcomes in critically ill adults. Cochrane Database Syst Rev 2015;(8):CD008875.

34. Bilimoria KY, Liu Y, Paruch JL, et al. Development and evaluation of the universal ACS NSQIP surgical risk calculator: a decision aid and informed consent tool for patients and surgeons. J Am Coll Surg 2013;217(5):833–42.e3.

35. Cullen S. Gastrostomy tube feeding in adults: the risks, benefits and alternatives. Proc Nutr Soc 2011;70(3):293–8.

36. Metheny NA, Meert KL, Clouse RE. Complications related to feeding tube placement. Curr Opin Gastroenterol 2007;23(2):178–82.

37. Poulose BK, Kaiser J, Beck WC, et al. Disease-based mortality after percutaneous endoscopic gastrostomy: utility of the enterprise data warehouse. Surg Endosc 2013;27(11):4119–23.

38. Grant DG, Bradley PT, Pothier DD, et al. Complications following gastrostomy tube insertion in patients with head and neck cancer: a prospective multi-

institution study, systematic review and meta-analysis. Clin Otolaryngol 2009; 34(2):103–12.

39. Wollman B, D'Agostino HB, Walus-Wigle JR, et al. Radiologic, endoscopic, and surgical gastrostomy: an institutional evaluation and meta-analysis of the literature. Radiology 1995;197(3):699–704.

40. Mansoor H, Masood MA, Yusuf MA. Complications of percutaneous endoscopic gastrostomy tube insertion in cancer patients: a retrospective study. J Gastrointest Cancer 2014;45(4):452–9.

41. Mizrahi I, Garg M, Divino CM, et al. Comparison of laparoscopic versus open approach to gastrostomy tubes. JSLS 2014;18(1):28–33.

42. Choi AH, O'Leary MP, Merchant SJ, et al. Complications of feeding jejunostomy tubes in patients with gastroesophageal cancer. J Gastrointest Surg 2017; 21(2):259–65.

43. Haskins IN, Strong AT, Baginsky M, et al. Comparison of laparoscopic jejunostomy tube to percutaneous endoscopic gastrostomy tube with jejunal extension: long-term durability and nutritional outcomes. Surg Endosc 2018;32(5): 2496–504.

44. Ukleja A, Romano MM. Complications of parenteral nutrition. Gastroenterol Clin North Am 2007;36(1):23–46.

45. Sowerbutts AM, Lal S, Sremanakova J, et al. Home parenteral nutrition for people with inoperable malignant bowel obstruction. Cochrane Database Syst Rev 2018;(8):CD012812.

46. Bozzetti F, Mariani L, Bertinet DB, et al. Central venous catheter complications in 447 patients on home parenteral nutrition: an analysis of over 100.000 catheter days. Clin Nutr 2002;21(6):475–85.

47. Moureau N, Poole S, Murdock MA, et al. Central venous catheters in home infusion care: outcomes analysis in 50,470 patients. J Vasc Interv Radiol 2002; 13(10):1009–16.

48. Plauth M, Cabré E, Campillo B, et al. ESPEN guidelines on parenteral nutrition: hepatology. Clin Nutr 2009;28(4):436–44.

49. Cano NJ, Aparicio M, Brunori G, et al. ESPEN guidelines on parenteral nutrition: adult renal failure. Clin Nutr 2009;28(4):401–14.

50. Oh SY, Jun HJ, Park SJ, et al. A randomized phase II study to assess the effectiveness of fluid therapy or intensive nutritional support on survival in patients with advanced cancer who cannot be nourished via enteral route. J Palliat Med 2014; 17(11):1266–70.

51. Bozzetti F. The role of parenteral nutrition in patients with malignant bowel obstruction. Support Care Cancer 2019;27(12):4393–9.

52. Nugent B, Lewis S, O'Sullivan JM. Enteral feeding methods for nutritional management in patients with head and neck cancers being treated with radiotherapy and/or chemotherapy. Cochrane Database Syst Rev 2013;(1):CD007904.

53. Baschnagel AM, Yadav S, Marina O, et al. Toxicities and costs of placing prophylactic and reactive percutaneous gastrostomy tubes in patients with locally advanced head and neck cancers treated with chemoradiotherapy. Head Neck 2014;36(8):1155–61.

54. Koretz RL, Lipman TO, Klein S. AGA technical review on parenteral nutrition. Gastroenterology 2001;121(4):970–1001.

55. Cotogni P, Monge T, Fadda M, et al. Bioelectrical impedance analysis for monitoring cancer patients receiving chemotherapy and home parenteral nutrition. BMC Cancer 2018;18(1):990.

56. Orrevall Y, Tishelman C, Permert J. Home parenteral nutrition: a qualitative interview study of the experiences of advanced cancer patients and their families. Clin Nutr 2005;24(6):961–70.

57. Keung EZ, Liu X, Nuzhad A, et al. In-hospital and long-term outcomes after percutaneous endoscopic gastrostomy in patients with malignancy. J Am Coll Surg 2012;215(6):777–86.

58. Richards DM, Tanikella R, Arora G, et al. Percutaneous endoscopic gastrostomy in cancer patients: predictors of 30-day complications, 30-day mortality, and overall mortality. Dig Dis Sci 2013;58(3):768–76.

59. Yost KJ, Thompson CA, Eton DT, et al. The Functional Assessment of Cancer Therapy - General (FACT-G) is valid for monitoring quality of life in patients with non-Hodgkin lymphoma. Leuk Lymphoma 2013;54(2):290–7.

60. Culine S, Chambrier C, Tadmouri A, et al. Home parenteral nutrition improves quality of life and nutritional status in patients with cancer: a French observational multicentre study. Support Care Cancer 2014;22(7):1867–74.

61. Bozzetti F, Cozzaglio L, Biganzoli E, et al. Quality of life and length of survival in advanced cancer patients on home parenteral nutrition. Clin Nutr 2002;21(4): 281–8.

62. Naghibi M, Smith TR, Elia M. A systematic review with meta-analysis of survival, quality of life and cost-effectiveness of home parenteral nutrition in patients with inoperable malignant bowel obstruction. Clin Nutr 2015;34(5):825–37.

63. Bozzetti F, Arends J, Lundholm K, et al. ESPEN guidelines on parenteral nutrition: non-surgical oncology. Clin Nutr 2009;28(4):445–54.

64. Ruggeri E, Giannantonio M, Agostini F, et al. Home artificial nutrition in palliative care cancer patients: impact on survival and performance status. Clin Nutr 2020; 39(11):3346–53.

65. Whitney SN, McGuire AL, McCullough LB. A typology of shared decision making, informed consent, and simple consent. Ann Intern Med 2004;140(1):54–9.

66. Druml C, Ballmer PE, Druml W, et al. ESPEN guideline on ethical aspects of artificial nutrition and hydration. Clin Nutr 2016;35(3):545–56.

Strategies for Optimizing Perioperative Pain Management for the Cancer Patient

Breana L. Hill, MD[a],*, Carolyn Lefkowits, MD[b]

KEYWORDS

- Cancer pain • Pain management • Total pain • Postoperative pain

KEY POINTS

- Acute postoperative pain in a patient with cancer must be distinguished and managed differently from chronic cancer-related pain.
- "Total pain" is an important concept that underscores the importance of a biopsychosocial approach to the management of pain in patients with cancer.
- Management of acute postoperative pain starts with education and expectation setting in the preoperative period.
- A multimodal approach to perioperative pain management should be used whenever possible.
- Surgeons must be mindful of the risk of new persistent opioid use developing in the postoperative period.

INTRODUCTION

Background

Pain in the population of patients with cancer is unique. It is characterized by multimorphism: by a physical nature classified by etiology, temporality, location, and time and by a psychological nature, with emotional, cognitive, and behavioral factors that impact pain. Psychological factors may increase the perception of pain, whereas improper pain control may also trigger psychological distress.[1] Pain syndromes in the patient with cancer can be broken down into those arising from the direct effect of neoplasm on nearby tissues (85%), the side effects of a cancer treatment (17%), disease progression (9%), and other causes not directly related to malignancy.[2] The

Financial Disclosures: The authors have nothing to disclose.
[a] Department of Obstetrics and Gynecology, University of Colorado School of Medicine, Aurora, CO, USA; [b] Department of Obstetrics and Gynecology, Division of Gynecologic Oncology, University of Colorado School of Medicine, Aurora, CO, USA
* Corresponding author. 12631 East 17th Avenue, B198-6, Aurora, CO 80045.
E-mail address: Breana.hill@cuanschutz.edu

Surg Oncol Clin N Am 30 (2021) 519–534
https://doi.org/10.1016/j.soc.2021.02.011
1055-3207/21/© 2021 Elsevier Inc. All rights reserved.

surgonc.theclinics.com

etiology of pain in a patient with cancer may vary at any given moment, from cancer-related chronic pain to acute surgical pain. Acute surgical pain may have some overlapping characteristics with chronic cancer pain. However, distinguishing these two is important, as the difference in expected chronicity impacts treatment strategies. We focus on management of acute surgical pain in the patient with cancer.

Prevalence

Pain impacts a large proportion of our population of patients with cancer. Pain prevalence averages 53% across the cancer continuum, from diagnosis through survivorship or end of life, and 38% of those patients define their pain as moderate to severe pain.[3,4] Chronic postsurgical pain, defined as pain related to a procedure persisting more than 2 to 3 months after surgery, continues to increase in the population of patients with cancer as survival outcomes improve.[5] The concept of "total pain" is an important one as it relates to the population of patients with cancer. "Total pain" includes sources of pain that are nonphysical (anxiety, rage, depression, interpersonal interactions, family strains, nonacceptance of caregivers, doubting faith, sense of hopelessness) and underscores the importance of a biopsychosocial approach to the management of pain in patients with cancer, whether it is acute postoperative pain or chronic cancer-related pain.[6]

Clinical Impact of Cancer-Related Pain

Proper management of cancer pain impacts our patients' quality of life and willingness to receive other disease-directed therapy.[3] One-sixth of patients with cancer have depression and one-quarter have other mood disorders while actively receiving treatment for their cancer. Major depression is associated not only with pain but also with a decrease in adherence to treatment, longer hospital stays, and increased suicide rates in patients with cancer.[3] The perioperative period is characterized by the surgical stress response, angiogenesis, and immunomodulation that may support tumor spread.[7] It has been suggested that managing pain in the immediate perioperative period provides an opportunity to modulate the consequences of the stress response on the immune system and potentially mitigate cancer spread.[7] Pain also has important socioeconomic implications, with increased health care costs and decreased productivity.[8]

This review focuses on preoperative, intraoperative, and postoperative strategies for management of perioperative pain in the patient with cancer, with specific attention to approaches centered on optimizing quality of life. We conclude by addressing pain in special populations, including patients with preoperative opioid use and those with a history of substance abuse, as well as pain control near the end of life.

PREOPERATIVE PAIN MANAGEMENT OF THE PATIENT WITH CANCER

Understanding mechanisms of cancer-related pain and expectation setting are integral to preoperative counseling with patients. Mechanisms of cancer-related pain likely include tissue destruction from tumor production of proteases, stimulation of cytokine secretion, and immune cell migration and nerve growth by substances produced by cancer cells. Once this occurs, it is thought that neuromodulators are released, leading to sensitization and activation of peripheral neurons, and overexpression of nociceptive mediators in the spinal cord. The result is increased pain signaling in patients with cancer.[9] Pain, however, is not necessarily proportional to tumor burden. It therefore must be understood by the patients that surgery with the objective of reducing (or even completely resecting) cancer burden may not resolve or even necessarily improve their pain. Moreover, as discussed in the introduction, total pain involves physical, psychological, and social components that are best addressed by a multidisciplinary approach with multimodal treatment strategies that should be initiated in the preoperative period.

Preoperative education that is age-appropriate and considers the individual patient's health literacy, cultural and linguistic competency, and allows adequate time for questions, should underscore the goals of postoperative pain management.[10] The idea of focusing on function when assessing postoperative pain management should be introduced preoperatively. Patients should be counseled, depending on the planned surgery, that they are unlikely to be pain free in the early postoperative period, and that the goal will be to keep the pain tolerable enough that it is not interfering with their function, particularly with respect to the things they need to do to recover (like sleep, eat, and ambulate). Individually tailored education programs for patients with increased needs (including medical comorbidities) are associated with reduced postoperative opioid consumption, less preoperative anxiety, fewer requests for sedatives, and reduced length of stay after surgery.[10] Special attention also must be given to those with opioid consumption before surgery, as addressed in the special populations section later in this article.

Preoperative evaluation including a detailed history of the patient's medical and psychiatric comorbidities, medications, and history of chronic pain, substance abuse, and previous postoperative responses to pain management will also help guide the postoperative pain management planning.[10]

INTRAOPERATIVE PAIN MANAGEMENT OF THE PATIENT WITH CANCER
Approach

Although intraoperative pain management is primarily the purview of our anesthesia colleagues, it behooves the surgeon to have some degree of familiarity with modalities used that help reduce postoperative nausea and vomiting, length of stay, and intensity of pain that might contribute to higher volume opioid consumption.[11]

Comprehensive coverage of Enhanced Recovery After Surgery (ERAS) protocols and their clinical impact is beyond the scope of this review but it should be noted that ERAS, although not unique to the population of patients with cancer, has resulted in shorter length of hospital stays, reductions in complications, and reduced readmissions and hospital costs.[12] Implementation of ERAS protocols have improved outcomes in almost all major surgical specialties and should be considered in the provider's approach to managing perioperative pain in the patient with cancer.

Pharmacologic Interventions

Modalities to improve perioperative pain control in the intraoperative setting include use of regional anesthesia, use of opioid-sparing anesthesia (including nerve blocks), balancing fluids, and maintaining temperature control. The emphasis of ERAS is on maintaining homeostasis and reducing the stress response.[12]

Several nerve blocks have been used by anesthesiologists, which depending on the procedure, might include thoracic paravertebral nerve block, transversus abdominis plane block, quadratus lumborum block, or neuraxial neurolytic blocks. Neuraxial neurolysis provides analgesia by blocking sensory fibers (A-delta and C-fibers) while preserving motor fibers, which serves patients with cancer willing to participate in physical rehabilitation especially well.[13] Intrathecal morphine was evaluated in a meta-analysis and concluded that it decreases pain intensity at rest and on movement up to 24 hours after major surgery.[14]

POSTOPERATIVE PAIN MANAGEMENT OF THE PATIENT WITH CANCER
Mechanisms and Risks of Chronic Postoperative Pain

The goal postoperatively is to return patients to their preoperative state of pain, if not better. Effectively managing postoperative pain requires an understanding of the pathophysiology and the potential for transition from acute to chronic pain.

Surgical trauma causes damage and inflammation, which leads to peripheral and then central sensitization. First, the surgical trauma activates and sensitizes C and A-δ fibers in the periphery, which releases glutamate and increases expression of sodium channels. Glutamate then activates iGlu (ligand-gated ionotropic receptors) and mGlu (G-protein couple metabotropic receptors). The progression from acute to chronic postsurgical pain may result from the activation of these iGlu receptors.[5] The exact mechanisms of postsurgical pain are not fully understood, and other suggested mechanisms involve pathophysiological changes related to long-term potentiation, activated microglial cells and astrocytes, chemokines, toll-like receptor 4 upregulation, increased spontaneous impulse discharges, reduced thresholds, loss of GABAergic descending modulation, protein kinase mediation, and expression of cathepsin G as a pronociceptive mediator.[5]

There are many risk factors for the development of chronic postsurgical pain (pain that persists for more than 2–3 months following surgery).[5] Preoperative pain and poorly managed acute perioperative pain are the 2 risk factors with the strongest correlation. Other risk factors include younger age, body mass index greater than 30, lower education level, type of surgery (with thoracotomy, breast, amputation, and hernia having higher associations), and chemotherapy and/or radiotherapy at any point during cancer treatment.[5] Considering total pain, psychological factors such as anxiety, depression, posttraumatic stress disorder, recall of perioperative pain, emotional function, and vulnerability all place a patient at higher risk of chronic postsurgical pain. Protective factors may include marriage, full-time employment, alcohol consumption, and cigarette smoking but their real effects remain unclear.[5]

Postoperative Pain Assessment

Pain assessment should be comprehensive and include pain characteristics, mechanisms, location, current analgesic treatment, and impact on function. Validated pain intensity assessment scales include the numerical rating scale, verbal rating scale, visual analog score, pain thermometer, and faces rating scale. However, postoperative pain assessment should not rely too heavily on pain intensity assessment scales because cancer pain is a multidimensional experience.[15] Judgment of adequacy of pain control should at least include, if not focus primarily on, impact of pain on function and ability to recover from surgery.

Pharmacologic Interventions

There is significant overlap in the pharmacologic modalities used for acute perioperative pain and chronic cancer-related pain. However, it is critical to maintain a distinction between the two when making a pain management plan, as the chronicity of the two differ, as does the role of opioids and appropriateness of long-term opioid use. Although a familiarity with some tenants of chronic cancer pain management may help the surgeon contextualize preoperative cancer-related pain, this section focuses on the management of acute surgical pain with the goal of returning the patient to their preoperative baseline (in terms of both pain and pain medication use). Medications used in the postoperative setting and their efficacies are briefly discussed here, with doses listed in **Table 1**.

Table 1
Medications with route of administration and dosing

Medication	Route of Administration	Starting Dose	Titration
Ibuprofen[52]	Oral, IV	Oral: 200–800 mg 3–4 times daily IV: 400–800 mg every 6 h PRN	Max dose: 3200 mg/d
Paracetamol[52]	Oral, IV, Rectal	Oral: 325–650 mg q4-6h or 1g q6h PRN IV: 650 mg q4h or 1g q6h Rectal: 325–650 mg q4–6h PRN	Max dose: 4 g/d Rectal max dose: 3.9 g/d
Morphine[53]	Oral, IV, IM (not recommended), Rectal, PCA	Oral: 10 mg q4h IV: 1 to 4 mg q1–4h PRN Rectal: 10 mg q4h PCA: 0.5 to 2 mg q5–10m	Oral: up to 30 mg q4h PRN IV: up to 10 mg q4h PRN PCA: Max dose 7.5 mg in 1 h, or 30 mg over a 4-h period
Oxycodone IR[54]	Oral, Rectal	Oral: 5–15 mg q4-6h Rectal: one suppository 3–4 times QD PRN	Titrate to appropriate effect
Oxycodone ER[54]	Oral	Oral tablet: 10 mg q12 h Oral capsules: 9 mg q12 h	Adjust dose in increments (25% to 50%) no more frequently than q1–2d (max 288 mg/d)
Hydrocodone[55]	Oral	Oral: 20 mg QD Zohydro: 10 mg q12 h	Increase 10–20 mg q3–5d Zohydro: 10 mg q12 h q3–7d ≥80 mg only in pts who are opioid tolerant
Hydromorphone[56]	Oral, IV, IM (not recommended), SubQ, PCA	Oral: 2 to 4 mg q4–6h PRN (tablets) or 2.5–10 mg q3–6h PRN (oral solution) IV: 0.2 mg to 1 mg q2–3h PRN SubQ: 1 to 2 mg q2–3h PRN PCA: Demand dose 0.1–0.4 mg q10 m	Titrate higher end of ranges for desired effect, opioid-tolerant patient may need higher initial dosing
Gabapentin[29]	Oral	300 mg to 1.2 g as single dose, 1–2 h before surgery or immediately following surgery	Prolonged use for neuropathic pain (range 300 mg TID to 1.2 g TID)
Pregabalin[29]	Oral	75–300 mg as single dose 1 h before surgery	Prolonged use for neuropathic pain (initial 25–150 mg/d in 2–3 divided doses, can increase 25–150 mg/d to a usual dose of 300–600 mg/d in 2–3 divided doses)

(continued on next page)

Table 1 (continued)			
Medication	Route of Administration	Starting Dose	Titration
Amitriptyline[31]	Oral	25 mg QHS (days −7 to −5 preoperatively), 50 mg QHS (days −4 to −3 preoperatively), 75 mg QHS (days −2 to −1 preoperatively)	N/A for surgical pain
Desipramine[31]	Oral	25 mg QHS (−7 to −5 preoperatively), then 50 mg QHS (days −4 to −3 preoperatively), 75 mg QHS (days −2 to −1 preoperatively)	N/A for surgical pain
Fluoxetine[31]	Oral	10 mg QHS for 7 d preoperatively	N/A for surgical pain
Lidocaine[34]	IV	10 mg or 1–3 mg/kg	Infusion of 1–5 µg/kg per h or 2-4 mg/min
Esmolol[35]	IV	Loading dose: 30–60 mg	Infusion of 5–500 µg/kg per min
Caffeine[36]	Oral	100–130 mg	N/A for surgical pain

Abbreviations: ER, extended release; IM, intramuscular; IR, immediate release; IV, intravenous; N/A, not applicable; PCA, patient-controlled analgesia; PRN, as needed; q, every; QD, every day; QHS, quaque hora somni (every evening); SubQ, subcutaneous; TID, 3 times a day.

Nonsteroidal anti-inflammatory drugs

Nonsteroidal anti-inflammatory drugs (NSAIDs) have been shown to function both peripherally and centrally in nociception by blocking prostaglandin production.[16] NSAIDs should be considered for all surgical procedures because they decrease opioid requirements, improve patient satisfaction, decrease recovery times, and decrease morbidity in the postoperative period.[16] A Cochrane review examined evidence for NSAIDs or paracetamol, alone or combined with opioids, in treating chronic cancer pain. The studies in the review were small and of poor quality, so the conclusion drawn was that the impact of using an NSAID alone for chronic cancer pain is unknown.[17] Despite the lack of evidence in specifically treating chronic cancer pain, NSAIDs should be used in managing postoperative pain in the patient with cancer.

Paracetamol (acetaminophen)

A review of 14 studies containing 1129 patients compared the efficacy of a combination of paracetamol with an NSAID, versus an NSAID alone in the acute postoperative period.[18] The review suggested that combining the two conferred additional pain control over either drug alone.[18] With regard to chronic cancer pain, a Cochrane review found no convincing evidence of paracetamol being different from placebo in improving quality of life, use of rescue medication, or participant satisfaction.[19] This supports the use of paracetamol in acute surgical pain, but not necessarily in chronic cancer pain.

Opioids

Opioids act by blocking pain receptors. Two commonly used opioids, morphine and oxycodone, act by blocking the μ receptor and κ receptor, respectively.[20] The oral bioavailability and potency of oxycodone is greater than that of morphine and has been shown to be more effective at blocking visceral pain, which may provide an added benefit when treating postsurgical pain.[20] A review of 26 clinical trials concluded that oral oxycodone had superior postoperative analgesic efficacy compared with placebo in patients undergoing a variety of surgeries, including laparoscopic cholecystectomy, abdominal or pelvic surgery, bunionectomy, breast surgery, and spine surgery.[20]

An individual approach should be implemented when prescribing opioids and should include whether the patient is opioid-naïve to determine the starting dose, frequency, and titration. The short half-life of opioid pure agonists (morphine, hydromorphone, fentanyl, and oxycodone) are preferred because they are easier to titrate than long half-life opioids (methadone, levorphanol).[21]

Persistent Opioid Use and Dose Reduction Postoperatively

Because surgery is an acute pain event, monitoring for postoperative opioid dose tapering should occur even in the population of patients with cancer. Opioids should be prescribed judiciously, with an understanding with the patient that the goal within a few weeks after surgery, is to have the patient return to his or her preoperative levels of opioid use (off opioids altogether if the patient was opioid-naïve at time of surgery). Opioids prescribed during and after surgery may beget long-term opioid use regardless of whether a patient is opioid tolerant or has had prior exposure to opioids.[22] More than 60% of people receiving 90 days of continuous opioid therapy postoperatively remain on opioids years later. Patients receiving an opioid prescription after short-stay surgeries have a 44% increased risk of long-term opioid use compared with those who did not receive an opioid prescription.[22] Measures to shorten duration of postoperative opioid use are necessary to limit the transition from acute to long-term opioid use.[22] Risk factors for chronic opioid use after surgery among opioid-naïve patients include male sex, age older than 50 years, preoperative use of benzodiazepines, preoperative use of antidepressants, depression history, and alcohol and drug abuse history.[22] Reduction of persistent opioid use involves multimodal analgesia (2 or more medications or nonpharmacologic interventions that often include gabapentinoids, acetaminophen, ketamine, NSAIDs, and regional anesthesia).[22] The standard of care is to advise patients to discontinue opioids when they no longer have pain, but a disconnect between opioids prescribed and opioids used after surgery exists, and patients usually self-taper with minimal instructions after surgery.[22]

Historically, physicians have overprescribed opioids. Alarmingly, 45% of patients who did not take opioids on their last day of surgical hospitalization were prescribed opioids at discharge.[23] Weston and colleagues[24] described a cohort of 108 patients who received a minimally invasive hysterectomy, in whom 79% had cancer. The median prescribed opioids were 30 pills, but median use was 10 pills. Mark and colleagues[25] performed a case-control study that included 1231 patients undergoing major gynecologic oncology surgery. The intervention group received an opioid-restrictive protocol, with patients prescribed no more than 3 days of opioids.[25] Mean opioid pill prescriptions went from 43.6 pills for open surgery and 38.4 pills for minimally invasive surgery to 12.1 and 1.3 pills, respectively. This intervention did not change postoperative pain scores, patient satisfaction, or refill requests, suggesting that a reduction in prescribed opioids is safe and attainable.[25]

New, persistent opioid use, defined as receiving an additional opioid prescription between 90 and 180 days after surgery, remains an issue in both the noncancer and cancer population postoperatively.[26] In a review of 68,463 patients undergoing curative-intent surgery who filled opioid prescriptions, 10.4% of opioid-naïve patients experienced new, persistent opioid use. One year after surgery, these patients continued to fill prescriptions to doses similar to chronic opioid users.[26]

Procedure-specific prescribing recommendations may help reduce the common overprescribing issue.[23] An expert panel consensus developed outpatient opioid prescribing ranges for 20 common surgical procedures in 8 surgical specialties, and although not specific to the cancer population, these may serve as a guideline in managing opioid prescriptions postoperatively.[23]

In addition to their time-limited role in postsurgical pain, according to the National Comprehensive Cancer Network (NCCN), opioids are one of the cornerstones of chronic cancer pain management.[21] The appropriate dose of opioid is based on the patient's pain intensity and treatment goals. The NCCN recommends considering opioid rotation (switching from one opioid to another) if pain is inadequately managed despite dose titration, or there are persistent adverse effects, change in condition (unable to tolerate oral medications), or restrictions due to cost or insurance coverage.[21]

Side effects of opioids are common and include constipation, nausea and vomiting, pruritus, delirium, respiratory depression, motor and cognitive impairment, and sedation. These side effects must be managed, as these physical symptoms can contribute to the total pain of the patient with cancer but also provide another reason to wean opioid use to that of the presurgical state.[27]

GABAPENTIN AND PREGABALIN

Gabapentin and pregabalin are both antiepileptics that bind to voltage-dependent calcium channels, which are found in the spinal cord. The action of these drugs inhibits the release of excitatory neurotransmitters and reduces glutamate availability at NMDA receptors. Pregabalin has analgesic, anxiolytic, and anticonvulsant activity and is 6 times more potent than gabapentin.[28] A review of the literature suggests that when neuropathic mechanisms of pain predominate, physicians should consider using a low-dose adjuvant, with the best evidence supporting use of gabapentin.[29] Their utility in postoperative pain and reduction of opioid consumption has also been researched, with numerous meta-analyses indicating their efficacy.[30] However, a more recent meta-analysis of 97 studies cautioned against their use given the risk of serious adverse events and only a modest opioid-sparing effect, and a different meta-analysis showed that pregabalin did not prevent development of chronic postsurgical pain.[30]

Observational studies have shown that neuropathic pain is found in 35.9% to 39.7% of patients with chronic cancer pain, suggesting that gabapentinoids can play a role in cancer pain separate from postsurgical pain.[29] Detailed discussion of gabapentinoid use for chronic cancer pain is outside the scope of this paper.

ANTIDEPRESSANTS

Tricyclic antidepressants, including amitriptyline and desipramine, are commonly used for various chronic pain conditions and have also been evaluated in a limited number of studies for acute postoperative pain. Only one study with amitriptyline showed significantly lower pain intensity at 24 hours postoperatively.[31] Desipramine showed promise when administered several days before surgery in 2 separate studies.[31] However, these studies were not specific to the patient with cancer and ultimately the limited evidence available does not support their use in the management of postoperative pain.[32]

Selective serotonin reuptake inhibitors and serotonin norepinephrine reuptake inhibitors were also evaluated for their clinical use in the postoperative setting. Fluoxetine showed no improvement over placebo in reducing opioid use.[31] In a group of patients undergoing mastectomy, venlafaxine was administered the evening before surgery and for the first 10 postoperative days. Pain with movement and use of postoperative analgesics were reduced in the venlafaxine group.[31] There remains limited available evidence to strongly suggest that duloxetine provides an opioid-sparing effect.[32]

LOCAL ANALGESICS

Lidocaine is commonly used for neuraxial and peripheral nerve blocks but also has analgesic properties when administered intravenously. Suggested mechanisms of action include decreased release of proinflammatory cytokines, nuclear factor-kB-modulated downregulation at the mRNA level, and inhibition of NMDA receptors.[33] A 2015 Cochrane review containing 43 randomized controlled trials compared intravenous lidocaine to placebo and concluded that a bolus of lidocaine (10 mg or 1 to 3 mg/kg), followed by an infusion (1 to 5 mg/kg per hour or 2 to 4 mg/min) reduced pain scores at 1 to 4 hours and 24 hours after surgery. It also decreased perioperative opioid requirements, decreased postoperative nausea, vomiting, and ileus, and shortened hospital length of stay by 8 hours.[34]

ESMOLOL

Esmolol is a selective β-1 blocker with rapid onset and offset. Given intravenously, its mechanisms of action in control of postoperative pain are speculative, but possibly include a blockade of the excitatory effects of pain signaling and modulation of central pronociceptive activity.[32] A meta-analysis concluded that perioperative infusion of esmolol (5–500 μg/kg per minute) with or without a loading dose resulted in lower pain scores, lower postoperative opioid consumption, and decreased postoperative nausea and vomiting. The meta-analysis did conclude that larger trials would need to be conducted given the high risk of bias in the studies reviewed.[35]

CAFFEINE

Caffeine is a methylxanthine, which acts as a central nervous system stimulant to increase wakefulness, endurance, heart rate, blood pressure, and mood.[36] Several studies have reviewed the effect of adding caffeine to analgesics, including paracetamol, aspirin, and ibuprofen for control of postsurgical pain. A Cochrane review recently evaluated 25 comparisons of analgesic plus caffeine versus analgesic alone in a total of 4262 participants.[36] The proportion of participants who achieved at least 50% pain relief was dose dependent: 6% at doses of 65 mg or less, 8% with doses between 70 and 150 mg, and 11% with doses of 150 mg or more. The review concluded that caffeine is effective at doses of 100 mg or more in providing pain relief for an additional 5% to 10% of patients. This was specifically evaluated in the postsurgical population, but little is known about its relief of chronic or nonsurgical pain.[36]

MEDICAL CANNABIS

Cannabinoids are commonly administered via inhalation, orally, or via sprays and have been suggested as modulators of the pain pathway through one of the body's endogenous signaling systems. A study containing 11 patients evaluated the impacts of dose escalation of cannabis extract (5, 10, or 15 mg) on postoperative pain.[37] Less rescue analgesia was requested, and pain intensity was decreased in the group that received 15 mg. However, these patients also experienced greater sedation, more adverse events, and the study was terminated early because of a serious vasovagal adverse event in a patient receiving 15 mg.[37] The study did conclude that the number needed to treat is equivalent to many routinely used analgesics without frequent adverse effects, but given the paucity of data, more research is needed before a recommendation for perioperative cannabis use can be made.

A review of 5 clinical studies evaluating the effects of cannabinoids on controlling cancer pain found evidence to suggest that medical cannabis use reduces chronic or neuropathic pain in patients with advanced cancer. The reviewers found that many of the studies lacked statistical power and concluded that there remains a need for further double-blind, placebo-controlled clinical trials with larger sample sizes to be able to establish optimal dosage and efficacy of cannabinoid therapy.[38]

SPECIAL POPULATIONS AND CIRCUMSTANCES
Patients with Preexisting Opioid Use

Inadequate pain management is common in patients with preexisting opioid use.[39] Patients taking opioids preoperatively have a higher risk of increased severity and duration of pain after surgery, prolonged postoperative opioid use, increased hospital length of stay, and postoperative complications. Providers must understand clinical phenomena that occur in patients with chronic opioid use, including tolerance, physical dependence, hyperalgesia, withdrawal, and addiction. Preoperative referral to an addiction specialist or to an acute pain service may also be warranted.[39]

Chronic opioid use causes central sensitization, which leads to increased severity of acute and chronic pain due to altering of signaling pathways. The preoperative evaluation should include differentiating between opioid use and abuse, evaluating for coexisting psychiatric disorders, avoiding biases, and gathering a comprehensive understanding of the patients' fears. There is insufficient evidence to decrease or discontinue opioids preoperatively, but it is helpful to develop a pain treatment plan.[39]

Several studies have suggested that opioid-dependent patients have fourfold increased opioid requirements in the postoperative period compared with those who are opioid-naïve.[40] Multimodal analgesia is particularly critical in these patients, including consideration of use of regional anesthesia and patient-controlled analgesia (PCAs). Advantages of PCAs in this patient population include maintaining stable plasma levels, pain relief with lower total opioid consumption, and fewer interactions between health care providers, which reduces patients' anxiety, prejudices, and acute withdrawal episodes.[40]

Ketamine is supported for postoperative pain control in opioid-tolerant patients.[41] Ketamine, by blocking NMDA receptors, can prevent central sensitization and inhibit wind-up phenomenon, opioid-related tolerance, hyperalgesia, and has shown improved pain control and reduction in opioid consumption postoperatively. There were no clear differences in adverse effects when using ketamine.[41] It may be helpful to involve anesthesia or pain specialist colleagues if considering ketamine use in patients with otherwise refractory perioperative pain.

Patients on methadone or buprenorphine require a different approach. For patients who present on these medications, involvement of anesthesia, pain, or addiction specialists beginning in the preoperative period is recommended where available. Daily doses of methadone should be continued with the addition of short-acting opioids and multimodal agents to manage the acute pain, while also considering the possibility of cross-tolerance.[42] Cross-tolerance may explain why patients on maintenance opioids often require higher and more frequent dosing of opioid analgesics. Analgesic dosing should be continuous to prevent reemergence of pain and reduce patient suffering and anxiety regarding adequate pain control. Mixed agonist/antagonist opioids should be avoided.[42] Buprenorphine, with its high affinity to the μ receptor, requires slightly more consideration with acute pain management. Options can include continuing maintenance therapy with titration of a short-acting opioid, dividing the dose of buprenorphine with administration every 6 to 8 hours, discontinuing buprenorphine, and treating the patient will full opioid agonist analgesics with titration to avoid withdrawal, or converting to methadone at 30 to 40 mg/d.[42] After treatment of acute pain, it should be kept in mind that a buprenorphine restart can precipitate opioid withdrawal.[42]

Pain Control in Presence of Substance Use Disorder

Substance use disorder is a common problem; it is a complex condition characterized by compulsion and preoccupation with a substance despite negative consequences. Patients with substance use disorder, like opioid-tolerant patients, may be at risk of having their acute pain undertreated related to their preexisting opioid tolerance, fears of precipitating respiratory depression and fears of triggering relapse.[43]

Providers may also fear inducing relapse. Patients with inadequate pain control, however, are more likely to self-medicate.[43] Providers should avoid using less potent opioids for this reason. The use of objective findings and specific pain complaints should provide the clinician with reassurance that the patient is not drug-seeking, which is a common prejudgment. Drug abuse screening tools and multimodal anesthesia should be used, but more research is needed to improve treatments for optimal pain relief and to prevent central sensitization, chronic pain, and impaired physical and social functioning in this patient population.[43]

Pain Control for Patients near the End of Life

The patient with cancer may be faced with significant pain at the end of life from a variety of causes, including tumor burden, surgical procedures, or other components of total pain. Barriers to pain control at the end of life include patient factors, clinician factors, family factors, and system factors. Patient factors may include the misconception of a dichotomous choice of being awake and in pain versus having pain controlled and being sedated, may fear the stigma of addiction, and might want to avoid opioid-related side effects. Clinicians may fear the inability to adequately recognize pain, may fear hastening death (although protected by the doctrine of double effect) and must deal with the competing goals of providing cure versus comfort. Family factors include desire for the patient to be alert and the fear of hastening death. System factors include fragmented care and medicolegal concerns regarding opioid prescribing.[44]

Three aspects of "a good death" have been previously described and include the following: avoidance of distress and suffering, alliance with patient's preferences and wishes, and consistence with clinical and cultural standards.[45] Pain control and patient comfort should be achieved at the end of life, with involvement of palliative care clinicians when beyond the scope of the surgeon.

NONPHARMACOLOGIC STRATEGIES

Nonpharmacologic strategies can be key elements in multimodal pain control. Although the data are limited, this section provides a brief review of some nonpharmacologic modalities used in the general postoperative setting, as well as in the management of chronic cancer pain.

Cognitive Behavioral Therapy

Cognitive behavioral therapy (CBT) is a form of psychotherapy that has been shown to relieve distress and pain in various cancer populations.[46] Hypnosis, a commonly used

CBT technique, has also been evaluated in the acute postsurgical setting. A meta-analysis indicated that hypnosis treatment groups had better outcomes than 89% of patients in control groups. In this nonpharmacologic intervention, a hypnotist guides a patient through peaceful and relaxing imagery in the induction phase to allow the patient to feel more relaxed, less distracted, and more open to therapeutic suggestions. In the application phase, the hypnotist makes suggestions for the patient to change sensorial or cognitive processes, physiology, or behavior. Hypnosis as an adjunct to postoperative pain control may be a powerful tool in addressing symptoms after surgery.[47]

Acupuncture

Acupuncture originated in Chinese medicine and involves the insertion of needles to defined depths, followed by manipulation with forces, heat, or electrical stimuli. A systematic review and meta-analysis found that patients treated with acupuncture or related techniques had less pain and used less opioid analgesics on the first day after surgery compared with controls.[48] Few randomized controlled trials have been conducted to evaluate acupuncture for cancer-related pain but contained small sample sizes, heterogeneous cancer diagnoses, and differing study methodologies. No definitive conclusion has been made to recommend acupuncture as part of standard care for treating cancer pain, but can continue to be used for postsurgical pain.[49]

Exercise

Prehabilitation training is the process of optimizing physical functionality before surgery and can include a combination of aerobic exercises, strength training, and functional task training.[50] A systematic review evaluated its utility in function, pain, and quality of life following surgery. They concluded that there was no benefit to pain, quality of life, readmissions or nursing home placement, but there was a significant reduction in the need for postoperative rehabilitation.[50]

Mishra and colleagues[51] conducted a Cochrane review containing 40 trials testing exercise interventions on quality of life for cancer survivors. Their results suggested that exercise compared with control has a positive impact on global health-related quality of life, body image/self-esteem, emotional well-being, sexuality, sleep disturbance, and social functioning. They also found that exercise interventions decreased anxiety, fatigue, and pain at 12 weeks' follow-up. They do mention that all trials reviewed were at high risk for performance bias and results should be interpreted cautiously.[51] Given the impact of total pain on the patient with cancer, exercise should still be considered as a nonpharmacologic option to control pain long after surgery. Additional research with focus on exercise and its impact specifically on cancer and postsurgical pain is needed.

DISCUSSION AND FUTURE DIRECTIONS

Pain is highly prevalent in the population of patients with cancer and spans from diagnosis through survivorship. Given the complexity of cancer pain, a multimodal approach is essential in managing perioperative pain. Chronic postsurgical pain continues to increase as survival outcomes improve, and the concept of total pain underscores the importance of managing more than just physical pain. Pain management begins in the preoperative setting, with the focus on patient education and expectation setting. Intraoperatively, anesthesia plays an important role in helping reduce postoperative nausea and vomiting, length of stay, and pain intensity. Management of postoperative pain should focus on how the pain is impacting the patient's function and recovery and may include both pharmacologic and nonpharmacologic therapies. Future directions will involve a multidisciplinary approach and likely include the surgeon, pain specialists, and behavioral therapists. More research needs to be done to assess the true efficacies of many of the pharmacologic modalities. The responsibility of the surgeon is to assess all dimensions of their patients' pain so that the appropriate treatment may be sought.

CLINICS CARE POINTS

- Pain impacts a large proportion of the population of patients with cancer, averaging 53% across the cancer continuum, at any given point from diagnosis to survival.
- Cancer pain is characterized by multimorphism and "total pain" must be considered.
- The focus of preoperative discussion should be education and expectation setting.
- Anesthesia plays an important role in maintaining homeostasis and reducing the stress response intraoperatively.
- Opioids are a cornerstone of postoperative pain therapy, but risk of prolonged use is a concern in the population of patients with cancer.
- Postoperatively, multimodal therapy is important in reducing postoperative opioid consumption, but further research needs to be done to evaluate the optimal means of opioid discontinuation while still decreasing postoperative pain.

REFERENCES

1. Minello C, George B, Allano G, et al. Assessing cancer pain-the first step toward improving patients' quality of life. Support Care Cancer 2019;27(8):3095–104.
2. Grond S ZD, Diefenbach C, Radbruch L, et al. Assessment of cancer pain: a prospective evaluation in 2266 cancer patients referred to a pain service. Pain 1996; 64:107–14.
3. Syrjala KL, Hensen MP, Mendoza ME, et al. Psychological and behavioral approaches to cancer pain management. J Clin Oncol 2014;32(16):1703–11.
4. van den Beuken-van Everdingen MH, Hochstenbach LM, Jooseten EA, et al. Update on prevalence of pain in patients with cancer: systematic review and meta-analysis. J Pain Symptom Manage 2016;51(6):1070–90.e9.
5. Humble Sr, Varela N, Jayaweera A, et al. Chronic postsurgical pain and cancer: the catch of surviving the unsurvivable. Curr Opin Support Palliat Care 2018; 12(2):118–23.
6. Clark D. 'Total pain', disciplinary power and the body in the work of Cicely Saunders, 1958–1967. Soc Sci Med 1999;49(6):727–36.
7. Missair A, Cata JP, Votta-Velis G, et al. Impact of perioperative pain management on cancer recurrence: an ASRA/ESRA special article. Reg Anesth Pain Med 2019;44(1):13–28.
8. Gustavsson A, Bjorkman J, Ljungcrantz C, et al. Socio-economic burden of patients with a diagnosis related to chronic pain–register data of 840,000 Swedish patients. Eur J Pain 2012;16(2):289–99.
9. Hacker KE, Reynolds RK, Uppal S. Ongoing strategies and updates on pain management in gynecologic oncology patients. Gynecol Oncol 2018;149(2): 410–9.
10. Chou R, Gordon DB, de Leon-Casasola OA, et al. Management of postoperative pain: a clinical practice guideline from the American Pain Society, the American

Society of Regional Anesthesia and Pain Medicine, and the American Society of Anesthesiologists' Committee on Regional Anesthesia, Executive Committee, and Administrative Council. J Pain 2016;17(2):131–57.

11. Liu SS, Richman JM, Wu CL. A comparison of regional versus general anesthesia for ambulatory anesthesia: a meta-analysis of randomized controlled trials. Anesth Analg 2005;101:1634–42.

12. Ljungqvist O, Scott M, Fearon KC. Enhanced recovery after surgery: a review. JAMA Surg 2017;152(3):292–8.

13. Candido KD, Kusper TM, Knezevic NN. New cancer pain treatment options. Curr Pain Headache Rep 2017;21(2):12.

14. Meylan N, Lysakowski C, Tramèr MR. Benefit and risk of intrathecal morphine without local anaesthetic in patients undergoing major surgery: meta-analysis of randomized trials. Br J Anaesth 2009;102:156–67.

15. Liu WC, Zheng ZX, Tan KH, et al. Multidimensional treatment of cancer pain. Curr Oncol Rep 2017;19(2):10.

16. Gupta A, Bah M. NSAIDs in the treatment of postoperative pain. Curr Pain Headache Rep 2016;20(11):62.

17. Derry S, Wiffen PJ, Moore RA, et al. Oral nonsteroidal anti-inflammatory drugs (NSAIDs) for cancer pain in adults. Cochrane Database Syst Rev 2017;(7): CD012638.

18. Ong CK, Seymour RA, Lirk P, et al. Combining paracetamol (acetaminophen) with nonsteroidal antiinflammatory drugs: a qualitative systematic review of analgesic efficacy for acute postoperative pain. Anesth Analg 2010;110(4):1170–9.

19. Wiffen PJ, Derry S, Moore RA, et al. Oral paracetamol (acetaminophen) for cancer pain. Cochrane Database Syst Rev 2017;(7):CD012637.

20. Cheung CW, Ching Wong SS, Qiu Q, et al. Oral oxycodone for acute postoperative pain: a review of clinical trials. Pain Physician 2017;20(2s):Se33–52.

21. NCCN. Clinical practice guidelines in oncology, adult cancer pain. 2017. Available at: https://www.nccn.org/professionals/physician_gls/pdf/pain.pdf. Accessed September 27, 2020.

22. Hah JM, Bateman BT, Ratliff J, et al. Chronic opioid use after surgery: implications for perioperative management in the face of the opioid epidemic. Anesth Analg 2017;125(5):1733–40.

23. Overton HN, Hanna MN, Bruhn WE, et al. Opioid-prescribing guidelines for common surgical procedures: an expert panel consensus. J Am Coll Surg 2018; 227(4):411–8.

24. Weston E, Raker C, Huang D, et al. Opioid use after minimally invasive hysterectomy in gynecologic oncology patients. Gynecol Oncol 2019;155(1):119–25.

25. Mark J, Argentieri DM, Gutierrez CA, et al. Ultrarestrictive opioid prescription protocol for pain management after gynecologic and abdominal surgery. JAMA Netw Open 2018;1(8):e185452.

26. Lee JS, Hu HM, Edelman AL, et al. New persistent opioid use among patients with cancer after curative-intent surgery. J Clin Oncol 2017;35(36):4042–9.

27. McNicol E, Horowicz-Mehler N, Fish RA, et al. Management of opioid side effects in cancer-related and chronic noncancer pain: a systematic review. J Pain 2003; 4:231–56.

28. Mishra S, Bhatnagar S, Goyal GN, et al. A comparative efficacy of amitriptyline, gabapentin, and pregabalin in neuropathic cancer pain: a prospective randomized double-blind placebo-controlled study. Am J Hosp Palliat Med 2012;29(3): 177–82.

29. Bennett MI. Effectiveness of antiepileptic or antidepressant drugs when added to opioids for cancer pain: systematic review. Palliat Med 2011;25(5):553–9.
30. Mitra S, Carlyle D, Kodumudi G, et al. New advances in acute postoperative pain management. Curr Pain Headache Rep 2018;22(5):35.
31. Wong K, Phelan R, Kalso E, et al. Antidepressant drugs for prevention of acute and chronic postsurgical pain: early evidence and recommended future directions. Anesthesiology 2014;121(3):591–608.
32. Kumar K, Kirksey M, Duong S, et al. A review of opioid-sparing modalities in perioperative pain management: methods to decrease opioid use postoperatively. Anesth Analgesia 2017;125(5):1749–60.
33. Brinkrolf P. Systemic lidocaine in surgical procedures: effects beyond sodium channel blockade. Curr Opin Anaesthesiol 2014;27:420–5.
34. Kranke P, Jokinen J, Pace NL, et al. Continuous intravenous perioperative lidocaine infusion for postoperative pain and recovery. Cochrane Database Syst Rev 2015;(7):CD009642.
35. Watts R, Calvert M, Newcombe G, et al. The effect of perioperative esmolol on early postoperative pain: a systematic review and meta-analysis. J Anaesthesiol Clin Pharmacol 2017;33:28–39.
36. Derry CJ, Moore RA. Caffeine as an analgesic adjuvant for acute pain in adults. Cochrane Database Syst Rev 2014;CD009281.
37. Holdcroft A, Maze M, Dore C, et al. A multicenter dose-escalation study of the analgesic and adverse effects of an oral cannabis extract (Cannador) for postoperative pain management. Anesthesiology 2006;104(5):1040–6.
38. Blake A, Wan BA, Malek L, et al. A selective review of medical cannabis in cancer pain management. Ann Palliat Med 2017;6(Suppl 2):S215–22.
39. Coluzzi F, Cuomo A, Dauri M, et al. The challenge of perioperative pain management in opioid-tolerant patients. Ther Clin Risk Manag 2017;13:1163–73.
40. Richebé P. Perioperative pain management in the patient treated with opioids: continuing professional development. Can J Anesth 2009;56:969–81.
41. Brinck EC, Tiippana E, Heesen M, et al. Perioperative intravenous ketamine for acute postoperative pain in adults. Cochrane Database Syst Rev 2018;(12): CD012033.
42. Alford D, Compton P, Samet JH. Acute pain management for patients receiving maintenance methadone or buprenorphine therapy. Ann Intern Med 2006;144: 127–34.
43. Vadivelu N, Lumermann L, Zhu R, et al. Pain control in the presence of drug addiction. Curr Pain Headache Rep 2016;20(5):35.
44. Steinhauser K, Christakis NA, Clipp EC, et al. Factors considered important at the end of life by patients, family, physicians and other care providers. JAMA 2000; 284(19):2476–82.
45. Mularski RA, Puntillo K, Varkey B, et al. Pain management within the palliative and end-of-life care experience in the ICU. Chest 2009;135(5):1360–9.
46. Tatrow K. Cognitive behavioral therapy techniques for distress and pain in breast cancer patients: a meta-analysis. J Behav Med 2006;29:17–27.
47. Montgomery GH, David D, Winkel G, et al. The effectiveness of adjunctive hypnosis with surgical patients: a meta-analysis. Anesth Analg 2002;94(6): 1639–45, table of contents.
48. Wu MS, Chen KH, Chen IF, et al. The efficacy of acupuncture in post-operative pain management: a systematic review and meta-analysis. PLoS One 2016; 11(3):e0150367.

49. Deng G, Bao T, Mao JJ. Understanding the benefits of acupuncture treatment for cancer pain management. Oncology (Williston Park) 2018;32(6):310–6.

50. Cabilan CJ, Hines S, Munday J. The effectiveness of prehabilitation or preoperative exercise for surgical patients: a systematic review. JBI Database Syst Rev Implement Rep 2015;13(1):146–87.

51. Mishra SI, Scherer RW, Geigle PM, et al. Exercise interventions on health-related quality of life for cancer survivors. Cochrane Database Syst Rev 2012;(8):CD007566.

52. APS. APS, Principles of analgesic use. 7th edition. Glenview, IL: American Pain Society; 2016.

53. Mariano E. Management of acute perioperative pain 2019. Post TW: Available at: http://www.uptodate.com. Accessed September 27, 2020.

54. APS. A.P.S., Principles of analgesic use in the treatment of acute pain and cancer pain. 6th edition. Glenview, IL: American Pain Society; 2008.

55. Hydrocodone: drug information. Available at: https://www.uptodate.com/contents/hydrocodone-drug-information?search=hydrocodone. Accessed September 28, 2020.

56. Hydromorphone: drug information. Available at: https://www.uptodate.com/contents/hydromorphone-drug-information?search=hydromorphone&source=panel_search_result&selectedTitle=1~149&usage_type=panel&kp_tab=drug_general&display_rank=1#references. Accessed September 27, 2020.

Navigating Difficult Conversations

Breaking Bad News and Exploring Goals of Care in Surgical Patients

Elizabeth J. Lilley, MD, MPH[a,b,c,*]

KEYWORDS

- Communication • Surgical patients • Palliative care • Oncology
- Doctor-patient relationship • Ethics

KEY POINTS

- Effective communication between surgeons and patients is essential for achieving optimal patient outcomes and goal-concordant surgery.
- Difficult communications can be navigated using a structured approach to understand patients' views and addressing their concerns.
- Accepting patients' emotional reactions and responding with empathic statements helps patients feel supported and heard.

INTRODUCTION

Effective communication is essential to providing optimal patient care. In surgery, doctor-patient communication faces unique challenges due to the typically short duration of the relationship combined with the surgeon's need to rapidly earn a patient's confidence. Favorable patient perceptions of their surgeons' communication skills are associated with improved patient satisfaction with care and adherence to medical treatments.[1] As such, skillful communication is valuable for building trust in the doctor-patient relationship and has a crucial role in patient safety and outcomes. Nonetheless, surgeons receive little training on how to navigate high-stakes communications, including conversations about poor prognosis and planning care at the end of life.

In contrast with other medical specialties, where a physician recommends a course of treatment and the patient is able to choose whether or not to take the prescribed

a Center for Surgery and Public Health at Brigham and Women's Hospital, Boston, 75 Francis St, Boston, MA 02115, USA; b Department of Psychosocial Oncology and Palliative Care, Dana-Farber Cancer Institute, Boston, MA, USA; c Division of Palliative Care and Geriatric Medicine, Department of Medicine, Massachusetts General Hospital, Boston, MA, USA
* Corresponding author. Center for Surgery and Public Health at Brigham and Women's Hospital, Boston, 75 Francis St, Boston, MA 02115, USA.
E-mail address: elilley@bwh.harvard.edu

Surg Oncol Clin N Am 30 (2021) 535–543
https://doi.org/10.1016/j.soc.2021.02.010
1055-3207/21/© 2021 Elsevier Inc. All rights reserved.
surgonc.theclinics.com

medication, surgical patients quite literally place their bodies in their surgeons' hands. This vulnerable state can contribute to a power imbalance in the surgeon-patient relationship and requires patients to have tremendous trust in their surgeons. Surgeons regularly use communication as a vehicle to demonstrate mastery over their craft and create rapport with patients and their families. However, as surgeons build confidence, they must also convey risk, uncertainty, and describe poor outcomes, which can be a challenging balance. The coexistence of these conflicting tasks within a single conversation exemplifies the complexity of communication in surgery.

Although most surgeons consider themselves to be good communicators, assessments of surgeons' communication skills from their patients, nurses, and colleagues demonstrate that there is much room for improvement.[2–5] In particular, surgeons struggle with conveying empathy and addressing patients' concerns during difficult communications.[2] These shortcomings are most needed in conversations that involve breaking bad news and exploring seriously ill patients' goals of care. This article provides a basic framework for approaching communication as a skill for surgeons to master as well as a deeper analysis of techniques for breaking bad news and exploring goals of care.

COMMUNICATION AS SKILL

In surgical lore, "The Gentleman Surgeon" archetype is characterized by his or her respectful nature and caring bedside manner. Although demonstrating respect and care is vital, the belief that excellent communication can be achieved by innately having a "nice" bedside manner trivializes its importance and disregards that communication is indeed a procedure requiring a compilation of technical skills.[6] Similar to master surgeons, skilled communicators can make a challenging conversation seem effortless, but on further examination there is finely honed technique at work.

As all procedural skills, communication can be improved through training and practice. Prior work has demonstrated that communication skills training improves surgeons' self-reported confidence and preparedness for difficult conversations.[7] Furthermore, health care professionals who have completed communication skills training are more likely to elicit patient concerns and demonstrate empathy toward their patients during conversations.[8] These communication techniques are valued by patients and families.[1,9] There are numerous available guides to support communications about treatment decision-making,[10–14] delivering bad news,[13,15,16] and addressing goals of care.[13,16–18] All of these guides share many of the same general principles with components that mirror the phases of a surgical operation: preparation, exploration, the "critical steps," and closure. These steps, as well as techniques for responding to emotion, are summarized in the following section.

Preparation

At the outset, there is a necessary recognition that difficult communications can have an emotional toll on patients. High-stakes conversations, as all procedures, have potential risks and complications.[6] Consequently, the decision to pursue these communications should be reached mindfully, with consideration of the need for the conversation to take place, the appropriate timing, and the desired outcomes. Before the conversation, necessary information should be gathered so that the surgeon can provide his or her clinical expertise. This may involve reviewing medical records and test results as well as speaking with other members of the medical team. Doing this anticipatory work before the conversation with the patient will help surgeons respond to questions posed by the patient and family and allow the conversation to move forward. It is also helpful to ask the patient who else they would want to be included in the discussion (eg, family members, other clinicians). Choosing a private location for the meeting can help to minimize interruptions and distractions.

Exploration

Just as the surgeon chooses the point of an incision based on where the critical steps of the operation will occur, the conversation should be initiated with the goal in mind. A natural impulse is to recap the patient's long medical history. However, this can be confusing for patients and families to follow and may not be relevant to the current situation. Instead of starting with a recitation of facts, asking the patient or family to share their thoughts and understanding allows clinicians to align with them and start from where they are. A systematic review of communications sharing limited prognosis for patients with advanced illness found that patients and family members appreciated when clinicians asked them to share their own understanding from what they have been told and what they have observed and also inquired about their individual preferences for receiving information.[9] This step is also a diagnostic exercise that helps to identify gaps in patients' understanding that can pose barriers to communication. Starting the conversation by listening to the patient's beliefs and concerns and then directly responding to what they have shared demonstrates your respect for the patient and shows that you have heard them.

Critical Steps

The critical steps of the conversation depend on its purpose. In many instances, a single conversation will contain more than one critical step. For example, after sharing that a patient has a bowel obstruction caused by disease progression in the abdomen (breaking bad news), the natural next step may be to ask the patient about what matters most to them (exploring goals of care) in order to provide a recommendation for treatment (surgical decision-making). The specific examples of breaking bad news and exploring goals of care are discussed in further detail later in this article.

Responding to Emotion

Much like a surgeon anticipates and is prepared to respond to hemorrhage during a procedure, clinicians must be ready to engage with the reactions of patients and other stakeholders during challenging communications. Throughout difficult conversations, patients and family members often react with emotion. Recognizing emotional reactions, validating the patient's right to have their feelings, and responding with statements that demonstrate empathy can support patients and family members and help them to recover and continue the conversation; this can be accomplished using the NURSE acronym (**Table 1**).[14,18] By using NURSE statements, the clinician accepts the patient's emotional response and acknowledges that patient's emotions are valid and important without trying to immediately reassure, agree, or contradict the emotion.[18]

Closure

In closing the conversation, it can be helpful to summarize key points and set expectations for what the next steps will look like. This is also an opportunity to clarify the patient's viewpoint. If the conversation has included making a treatment decision, it can be helpful to have the patient repeat their understanding of the treatment back to you to ensure that they understand. After the conversation has ended, the final steps are to debrief with the team and document the discussion. Debriefing provides the team an opportunity to ensure a common understanding of the plan and provide

Table 1
The NURSE mnemonic is a helpful tool for responding to emotions and demonstrating empathy

	Example	Notes
Naming	"It sounds like you are frustrated"	In general, turn down the intensity a notch when you name the emotion
Understanding	"This helps me understand what you are thinking"	Think of this as another kind of acknowledgment but stop short of suggesting you understand everything (you don't)
Respecting	"I can see you have really been trying to follow our instructions"	Remember that praise also fits in here eg "I think you have done a great job with this"
Supporting	"I will do my best to make sure you have what you need"	Making this kind of commitment is a powerful statement
Exploring	"Could you say more about what you mean when you say that…"	Asking a focused question prevents this from seeming too obvious

Using these statements acknowledges the patients' emotions and provides a moment to reflect on the emotional reaction rather than immediately offering reassurance, agreement, or contradiction.

Adapted from VitalTalk. Responding to Emotion: Articulating empathy using NURSE statements. 2019; https://www.vitaltalk.org/guides/responding-to-emotion-respecting/. Accessed 09/15/2020, with permission.

feedback on what went well and what could be done differently in the future. Documentation in the medical record provides a record of the communication, which can be referenced by other clinicians to guide future conversations.

Breaking Bad News

Surgical oncologists are involved at both the beginning and end of patients' cancer trajectories. As such, they are tasked with a range of challenging conversations that involve sharing difficult news. Early in the disease trajectory, surgeons may be involved in making the initial cancer diagnosis, directing the workup for metastatic disease, and determining eligibility for curative resection or advising when surgery will not be possible due to unresectable disease or poor baseline health. Later in the disease course, surgeons are consulted for patients with metastatic disease suffering from burdensome complications of advanced malignancy as well as patients who experience emergent surgical conditions in the setting of toxic systemic therapy for cancer. In these scenarios, the patient's health trajectory is altered by the acute condition regardless of whether a high-risk, emergency operation is performed. Therefore, surgical decision-making occurs in the context of breaking bad news.[10,12,19]

Conversations involving disclosure of difficult news for patients who have experienced surgical complications are particularly fraught. Landmark ethnographic work by medical sociologist Charles Bosk described surgeons' heightened feelings of responsibility for their patients' poor outcomes.[20] Building on this, medical anthropologist Joan Cassell introduced the concept of a "surgical covenant" in which the surgeon pledges to do all within his or her power to keep the patient alive.[21] These aspects of the surgeon-patient relationship illustrate how complications can pose a threat to the surgeon identity, which is rooted in the pursuit of perfection of clinical judgment and technical skill. One study by Schwarze and colleagues[22] demonstrated that when surgeons felt direct responsibility for complications, they were less willing to accept family members' desire to withdraw life-sustaining treatment. This highlights the unconscious biases that surgeons may bring to these conversations and the potential impact on treatment decisions.

There are several structured communication models for delivering bad news. The GUIDE approach is depicted in **Table 2**. When delivering difficult news, it is helpful to give a "warning shot" sentence. Stating "I am afraid I have some challenging news to share" cues the patient and family of what is to come and allows a moment to prepare to receive the news. After the warning shot, deliver the news as a single headline sentence clearly and concisely and then pause so the patient and family can absorb the news and respond. If the initial reaction is an emotional response, it is important to acknowledge the emotion and address it, which can be done using NURSE statements.

When the patient and family seem ready to receive more information, the remainder of the news should be delivered in small pieces, being careful to avoid jargon. Important points may need to be repeated or clarified. Building in pauses after delivering each unit of information lets the patient and family process and respond to the news. Emotional arousal can impair memory and cognitive processing abilities,[23] so it may be necessary to provide time for cognitive recovery before moving on to discussing goals or decision-making about treatment.

Goals of Care

Although the term "goals of care conversation" is often associated with care near the end of life, eliciting and understanding patients' goals of care is beneficial for patients

Table 2	
The GUIDE mnemonic is a tool for breaking bad news	
Step	**What You Say or Do**
Get Ready – Info, People, Place	"Let me take a minute to make sure I've got what I need." Make sure you have all the information you need at hand. Make sure you have all the right people in the room. Find a place with some privacy.
Understand what the patient knows	"What thoughts have you had since the biopsy?" "What have you taken away from other doctors so far?"
Inform starting with a headline	"The CT scan shows that the cancer has gotten worse" Give the information clearly and to the point with a one-sentence headline of the most important piece of information you want them to take away. Avoid jargon After the headline you will need to give more information, but after giving the headline, STOP!
Demonstrate empathy Respond directly to emotion	"I can see this news is not what you were hoping for." Expect the patient's first response to be emotion. Acknowledge the emotion explicitly.
Equip the patient for the next step	"Is there anything I could do to make this a little easier?" "I want you to be prepared for the next step. Can I explain…" Don't dismiss concerns or say that everything will be fine.

These conversations should begin by eliciting the patient's illness understanding. After delivering the news as a headline, it is necessary to pause and allow the patient to absorb and respond before moving forward.

Adapted from VitalTalk. Serious News: Breaking bad news using the GUIDE tool. 2019; https://www.vitaltalk.org/topics/disclose-serious-news/. Accessed 09/01/2020, with permission.

at all phases of cancer treatment. Exploring patients' beliefs, preferences, and values before high-risk operations helps build a deeper understanding of whether treatments will help patients achieve these stated goals. It also empowers patients to state the limitations on what treatments would be acceptable to them, rather than assuming that patients will "buy-in" to postoperative life support if they experience complications.[24] Although patients' perspectives often change over the course of their disease, these early communications can lay a foundation for future conversations.

Conversations about goals of care are also beneficial before interventions with palliative intent or urgent and emergent operations with high likelihood of poor outcomes.[10,11,25–30] These conversations often will follow a disclosure of bad news or some acknowledgment that the clinical picture has changed (eg, "We are in a different place now"). In this context, the purpose of the conversation is to ensure that recommended surgical treatments and postoperative care will align with patients' stated preferences. Asking patients about what matters most to them creates a common reference point to measure the risks and benefits of different treatment options. The Serious Illness Conversation Guide, developed at Ariadne Labs, is depicted in **Table 3**.

Patients facing serious illness can have many different types of goals, including attending important milestone events, completing meaningful projects, and maintaining levels of functioning or independence. In addition, asking patients what they worry about with respect to their health allows them to share concerns about the future and gives clinicians key information that is likely to influence their decisions.

Discussing patients' perspectives on tradeoffs is particularly relevant in surgery, where the decision for intervention is accompanied by accepting risk, postoperative symptoms, and the potential for prolonged recovery with diminished quality of life.[31]

Table 3
The REMAP mnemonic is a tool to approach conversations exploring patients' goals of care

Step	What You Say or Do
Reframe why the status quo isn't working.	You may need to discuss serious news (e.g. a scan result) first. "Given this news, it seems like a good time to talk about what to do now." "We're in a different place."
Expect emotion & empathize.	"It's hard to deal with all this." "I can see you are really concerned about [x]." "Tell me more about that—what are you worried about?" "Is it ok for us to talk about what this means?"
Map the future.	"Given this situation, what's most important for you?" "When you think about the future, are there things you want to do?" "As you think towards the future, what concerns you?"
Align with the patient's values.	As I listen to you, it sounds the most important things are [x,y,z].
Plan medical treatments that match patient values.	Here's what I can do now that will help you do those important things. What do you think about it?

These communications will often follow a disclosure of bad news. When goals of care are being discussed early in the disease course, the focus can be on mapping the future to understand the patient's hopes and worries with regard to their disease.

Adapted from VitalTalk. Addressing Goals of Care: Using the REMAP tool. 2019; https://www.vitaltalk.org/topics/reset-goals-of-care/. Accessed 9/8/2020, with permission.

Knowing what patients would and would not be willing to go through for more time is useful information in determining whether a surgical procedure is appropriate. Summarizing and reciting these preferences back to patients lets patients know that you have understood their wishes and gives patients the opportunity to clarify or correct any misinterpretations.

Palliative Care: an Added Layer of Support

It is also important to remember that in challenging communications, as in surgery, occasional complications are unavoidable. Despite meticulous preparation and exceptional skills, there will be times when conflicts arise during these conversations or other factors render these conversations more challenging. Although all physicians should have basic skills for difficult communications, palliative care specialist consultations can and should be requested for instances where these conversations are more complex.

Palliative care uses an interdisciplinary team model that includes physicians, nurse practitioners, chaplains, and social workers to help meet the multifaceted needs of seriously ill patients. Palliative care clinicians receive specialized communication training, which equips them to support patients and their medical teams through complex communications. Examples of scenarios that could benefit from palliative care expertise include patients who are unable or unwilling to participate in decision-making, conflicts among family members with ambiguity surrounding who has decisional authority, and conflicts among team members with differing perspectives on the appropriateness of the treatment plan. In these situations, interdisciplinary palliative care teams can provide an added layer of support to teams and help to identify and address unmet psychosocial and spiritual needs.

Successfully navigating difficult communications with surgical patients and their families requires empathy as well as planning, skill, and knowledge of available resources. Practicing communication techniques and using a structured approach to difficult conversations can help patients feels supported and respected and strengthen the surgeon-patient relationship.

CLINICS CARE POINTS

- Prepare for the meeting by reviewing medical records and gathering important information from other members of the medical team.
- If having an interdisciplinary meeting, the clinical team should assemble before speaking with the patient to assign roles and outline the goals of the conversation.
- Start the conversation by exploring the patient's or family's understanding. This provides space for patients and families to share their perceptions and concerns.
- When sharing difficult news, provide the information in short headline sentences and then give time to process this information.
- Acknowledge and respond to emotion using NURSE statements.
- Summarize the key points of the conversation and set expectations for the next steps.
- Debrief after meetings with other members of the clinical team and document the conversation in the medical record.

DISCLOSURE

The author has nothing to disclose.

REFERENCES

1. Schmocker RK, Cherney Stafford LM, Siy AB, et al. Understanding the determinants of patient satisfaction with surgical care using the Consumer Assessment of Healthcare Providers and Systems surgical care survey (S-CAHPS). Surgery 2015;158(6):1724–33.
2. Levinson W, Hudak P, Tricco AC. A systematic review of surgeon-patient communication: strengths and opportunities for improvement. Patient Educ Couns 2013; 93(1):3–17.
3. Makary MA, Sexton JB, Freischlag JA, et al. Operating room teamwork among physicians and nurses: teamwork in the eye of the beholder. J Am Coll Surg 2006;202(5):746–52.
4. Wauben LS, Dekker-van Doorn CM, van Wijngaarden JD, et al. Discrepant perceptions of communication, teamwork and situation awareness among surgical team members. Int J Qual Health Care 2011;23(2):159–66.
5. Quigley DD, Elliott MN, Farley DO, et al. Specialties differ in which aspects of doctor communication predict overall physician ratings. J Gen Intern Med 2014;29(3):447–54.
6. Lakin JR, Tulsky JA, Bernacki RE. Time out before talking: communication as a medical procedure. Ann Intern Med 2021;174(1):96–7.
7. Nakagawa S, Fischkoff K, Berlin A, et al. Communication Skills Training for General Surgery Residents. J Surg Educ 2019;76(5):1223–30.
8. Moore PM, Rivera S, Bravo-Soto GA, et al. Communication skills training for healthcare professionals working with people who have cancer. Cochrane database Syst Rev 2018;7:CD003751.
9. Parker SM, Clayton JM, Hancock K, et al. A systematic review of prognostic/end-of-life communication with adults in the advanced stages of a life-limiting illness: patient/caregiver preferences for the content, style, and timing of information. J Pain Symptom Manage 2007;34(1):81–93.
10. Cooper Z, Koritsanszky LA, Cauley CE, et al. Recommendations for best communication practices to facilitate goal-concordant care for seriously Ill older patients with emergency surgical conditions. Ann Surg 2016;263(1):1–6.
11. Miner TJ, Cohen J, Charpentier K, et al. The palliative triangle: improved patient selection and outcomes associated with palliative operations. Arch Surg 2011; 146(5):517–22.
12. Taylor LJ, Nabozny MJ, Steffens NM, et al. A framework to improve surgeon communication in high-stakes surgical decisions: best case/worst case. JAMA Surg 2017;152(6):531–8.
13. Widera E, Anderson WG, Santhosh L, et al. Family meetings on behalf of patients with serious Illness. N Engl J Med 2020;383(11):e71.
14. VitalTalk. Responding to Emotion: Articulating empathy using NURSE statements. 2019. Available at: https://www.vitaltalk.org/guides/responding-to-emotion-respecting/. Accessed September 15, 2020.
15. VitalTalk. Serious News: Breaking bad news using the GUIDE tool. 2019. Available at: https://www.vitaltalk.org/topics/disclose-serious-news/. Accessed September 01, 2020.
16. AriadneLabs. Serious Illness care. Available at: https://www.ariadnelabs.org/areas-of-work/serious-illness-care/. Accessed September 04, 2020.
17. VitalTalk. Addressing Goals of care: using the REMAP tool. 2019. Available at: https://www.vitaltalk.org/topics/reset-goals-of-care/. Accessed September 8, 2020.

18. Back AL, Arnold RM, Baile WF, et al. Approaching difficult communication tasks in oncology. CA Cancer J Clin 2005;55(3):164–77.
19. Lilley EJ, Cauley CE, Cooper Z. Using a Palliative care framework for seriously Ill surgical patients: the example of malignant bowel obstruction. JAMA Surg 2016; 151(8):695–6.
20. Bosk CL. Forgive and remember: managing medical failure. Chicago: University of Chicago Press; 1979.
21. Cassell J, Buchman TG, Streat S, et al. Surgeons, intensivists, and the covenant of care: administrative models and values affecting care at the end of life–updated. Crit Care Med 2003;31(5):1551–7, discussion 1557-1559.
22. Schwarze ML, Redmann AJ, Brasel KJ, et al. The role of surgeon error in withdrawal of postoperative life support. Ann Surg 2012;256(1):10–5.
23. Schwabe L, Joels M, Roozendaal B, et al. Stress effects on memory: an update and integration. Neurosci Biobehav Rev 2012;36(7):1740–9.
24. Schwarze ML, Redmann AJ, Alexander GC, et al. Surgeons expect patients to buy-in to postoperative life support preoperatively: results of a national survey. Crit Care Med 2013;41(1):1–8.
25. Cooper Z, Corso K, Bernacki R, et al. Conversations about treatment preferences before high-risk surgery: a pilot study in the preoperative testing center. J Palliat Med 2014;17(6):701–7.
26. Cooper Z, Courtwright A, Karlage A, et al. Pitfalls in communication that lead to nonbeneficial emergency surgery in elderly patients with serious illness: description of the problem and elements of a solution. Ann Surg 2014;260(6):949–57.
27. Lilley EJ, Bader AM, Cooper Z. A values-based conceptual framework for surgical appropriateness: an illustrative case report. Ann Palliat Med 2015;4(2):54–7.
28. Lilley EJ, Lindvall C, Lillemoe KD, et al. Measuring processes of care in palliative surgery: a novel approach using natural language processing. Ann Surg 2018; 267(5):823–5.
29. Miner TJ. Communication skills in palliative surgery: skill and effort are key. Surg Clin North Am 2011;91(2):355–66, ix.
30. Schwarze ML, Kehler JM, Campbell TC. Navigating high risk procedures with more than just a street map. J Palliat Med 2013;16(10):1169–71.
31. Bernacki RE, Block SD. American College of Physicians High Value Care Task F. Communication about serious illness care goals: a review and synthesis of best practices. JAMA Intern Med 2014;174(12):1994–2003.

Palliative Chemotherapy and the Surgical Oncologist

Elizabeth Wulff-Burchfield, MD[a,b,c], Lori Spoozak, MD, MHS[d,e], Esmé Finlay, MD[f,*]

KEYWORDS

- Palliative chemotherapy • Advanced cancer • Shared decision-making

KEY POINTS

- The term palliative chemotherapy can encompass a wide range of systemic therapies and possible treatment outcomes for advanced cancer.
- Systemic cancer therapy is evolving rapidly, but some classes have established perioperative risks such as infection, venous thromboembolism, and impaired wound healing.
- When surgery is being considered for advanced cancer, collaborative communication is essential to determine the impacts of systemic cancer therapy on surgical risks and outcomes.
- Following a structured communication framework can ensure that all prognostic, pharmacologic, and surgical issues are incorporated into medical decision-making.

INTRODUCTION

Patients who receive systemic cancer treatments in the setting of advanced disease are often described as receiving palliative chemotherapy, but this term has become increasingly problematic as systemic cancer therapies and advanced cancer outcomes have improved. Now that patients are living longer with cancer as a chronic life-limiting illness, surgeons may be increasingly asked to consider operating on those receiving palliative systemic treatments. In this review, we consider the term palliative chemotherapy and contextualize it based on current treatment paradigms. To facilitate optimally coordinated care between surgical and medical oncologists, we will

[a] Division of Medical Oncology, University of Kansas Medical Center, Kansas City, KS, USA;
[b] Division of Palliative Medicine, University of Kansas Medical Center, Kansas City, KS, USA;
[c] The University of Kansas Medical Center, 2330 Shawnee Mission Pkwy, Mail Stop 5003, Westwood, KS 66205, USA; [d] Division of Gynecologic Oncology, University of Kansas Medical Center, 3901 Rainbow, MS 2028, Kansas City, KS 66160, USA; [e] Division of Palliative Medicine, University of Kansas Medical Center, 3901 Rainbow, MS 2028, Kansas City, KS 66160, USA; [f] Department of Internal Medicine, Division of Palliative Medicine, University of New Mexico School of Medicine, The University of New Mexico Health Sciences Center, MSC10 5550, 1 University of New Mexico, Albuquerque, NM 87131-0001, USA
* Corresponding author.
E-mail address: efinlay@salud.unm.edu

Surg Oncol Clin N Am 30 (2021) 545–561
https://doi.org/10.1016/j.soc.2021.02.008
1055-3207/21/© 2021 Elsevier Inc. All rights reserved.

briefly review evidence about perioperative risks associated with select classes of systemic cancer treatments frequently used to treat patients with advanced cancer, and guidelines that surgeons may consider when planning interventions for patients with advanced cancer who are receiving systemic palliative treatments. Finally, a case-based communication framework is provided to enhance perioperative communication between medical and surgical oncologists who are collaborating to care for patients receiving palliative chemotherapy.

BACKGROUND, DEFINITIONS, AND LEXICAL GAPS

Despite widespread use, the term palliative chemotherapy not been consistently defined within the medical community.[1–3] Attempts to refine this terminology[1,2,4] have not generated consensus on the most appropriate or accurate alternatives that integrate the nuanced clinical and prognostic landscape and expanding pharmacologic options for treatment of patients with advanced cancer. Case 1 A illustrates this point.

Case 1A

Jillian Jones is a 56-year-old woman with stage IV colon adenocarcinoma with an isolated liver metastasis. Her functional status is excellent, and she has no comorbidities. She is motivated to receive aggressive cancer treatment. After a tumor board discussion, her medical and surgical oncologists agree that she should be offered chemotherapy with 5-fluorouracil, leucovorin, and oxaliplatin (FOLFOX) with the hope that her disease will become resectable. Four cycles of FOLFOX are recommended to limit hepatotoxicity.

After chemotherapy, her cancer status is reevaluated. Her liver metastasis is now resectable and no new metastatic disease is identified. She is offered resection of her primary colon mass and her liver metastasis.

Question: Is this patient being treated with curative or palliative intent? In this case, was FOLFOX "palliative chemotherapy?"

The word palliative has been used variably in relation to systemic cancer treatments. In some instances, such as the administration of gemcitabine for metastatic pancreatic cancer,[5] palliative has been applied literally, indicating that the treatment was approved based on its ability to improve symptoms and quality of life. In other situations, palliative chemotherapy describes treatment given to patients with advanced cancer without curative intent, with a goal of controlling or shrinking tumors and extending a patient's life, regardless of symptomatic outcomes.[1–3] Given the lack of consensus within the medical community, it is no surprise that patients and providers lack clarity about the intent of palliative chemotherapy.[6]

Further confounding the meaning of palliative chemotherapy, palliative medicine consultation is now recommended concurrently with oncology care for patients with advanced cancer[7] owing to landmark studies demonstrating improved quality of life, mood, goal-concordant care, and other positive outcomes.[8–11] Therefore, patients with advanced cancer may receive both palliative care consultative services and palliative chemotherapy concomitantly. Some experts have suggested abandoning the term palliative chemotherapy in part to prevent patients, caregivers, and health care professionals conflating systemic cancer treatment with specialty palliative care.[2]

Chemotherapy was once a less ambiguous term in oncology, typically referring to conventional cytotoxic agents. Applying a broader definition, with chemotherapy encompassing "any chemical agent or drug[12]" used to treat cancer, systemic treatments with diverse mechanisms of action, including cytotoxic chemotherapies, endocrine therapies, targeted therapies, checkpoint inhibitors, and cytokine immuno-therapy, may all be labeled palliative chemotherapy and administered to people with advanced disease. In addition, with the rapid advancement in the diversity and efficacy of systemic therapies for advanced cancer treatment, survival outcomes have also changed, now occasionally blurring the line between curative and noncurative treatment intent.

Although some existing terminology creates a shared understanding between providers regarding the intent of a systemic cancer treatment (eg, adjuvant treatment after the resection of invasive ductal carcinoma of the breast), the expanding systemic treatment options for patients with advanced disease have left oncologists with a lexical gap. Palliative chemotherapy is no longer an accurate or specific enough term to describe all systemic, cancer-directed therapies administered without the expectation of cure. Until such a lexicon exists, direct communication regarding palliative chemotherapy treatment objectives should be incorporated into interdisciplinary discussions and between providers and patients when determining the plan of care.

COMMUNICATION FRAMEWORK ABOUT SYSTEMIC THERAPY FOR PATIENTS WITH ADVANCED CANCER

Surgical oncologists routinely undertake complex preoperative risk assessment and decision-making when considering operative intervention for a patient with advanced cancer, including the evaluation of performance status, nutritional state, comorbidities, and goals. If a patient may receive perioperative systemic cancer treatment, risk stratification should include a review of current and future disease-directed therapies to determine the impacts on surgical risk, timing, and anticipated recovery period. If a prolonged postoperative chemotherapeutic holiday is recommended, this factor may increase the risk of tumor progression. Interdisciplinary communication between surgical and medical oncologists, and with patients and families, helps to integrate information regarding systemic therapy into operative planning, and may inform timing and choice of systemic therapy. The topics discussed in this article can be used to inform discussions and decision making when patients with advanced cancer on systemic therapy require surgery.

Step 1: Prognostic considerations
- Undertake routine preoperative risk stratification regarding performance status, nutrition, and comorbidities.
- Establish prognosis with and without operative management.
- Establish prognosis related to further systemic treatment (eg, is further systemic therapy recommended? Would overall prognosis be negatively impacted if it were delayed or could not be resumed owing to surgical recovery?
- Apply prognostic nomograms specific to cancer type or surgery, if available.

Step 2: Patient goals and tolerance of medical burden
- Assess patient expectations regarding cancer outcomes and quality of life.
- Consider use of communication tools such as best case scenario/worst case scenario.[13]

Step 3: Surgical oncology considerations
- Clarify the intent of surgical intervention.
- Assess the urgency of surgery; optimize preoperative condition when feasible.

Step 4: Medical oncology considerations
- Clarify the intent of systemic treatment.
- Discuss perioperative risks associated with the current and/or planned systemic treatment, including infectious complications, wound healing, and hemostasis.

- Discuss the timing of perioperative systemic treatment in relation to surgery.
- If further systemic therapy is medically inappropriate, explore the prognostic implications.

Step 5: Palliative care considerations

- Consider palliative care consultation if:
  - Requested by the patient or family;
  - Patient's performance status or comorbidities preclude surgery or systemic cancer therapy;
  - Patient symptom burden is high; or
  - Patient goals require further clarification.

Step 6: Coordinated decision-making

- Align patient goals and treatment plan.
- Formalize plans for managing systemic cancer therapy preoperatively.
- Discuss postoperative supportive care and the timing of postoperative systemic treatment, if indicated.

In case 1A (**Table 1**), key questions remained regarding the intent of treatment based on its designation as palliative chemotherapy. When applied to this case, the communication framework assures that all domains have been addressed before surgical planning.

Case 1A Conclusion

Ms Jones' tumor responds to FOLFOX, and repeat imaging indicates that aggressive surgical management is appropriate. This plan is aligned with her goals of care, and plans are made for her to undergo 4 months of postoperative FOLFOX to receive a total course of 6 months of systemic treatment, beginning 1 month postoperatively. She completes these interventions and has a 3-year disease-free interval.

Using communication and a treatment planning framework, clinicians can overcome any perceived ambiguity associated with the term palliative chemotherapy associated with the treatment intent. Although there is no substitute for

Table 1	
Case 1A: Ms Jones presents with a new diagnosis of colon adenocarcinoma with liver metastasis	
Prognostic considerations	Eastern Cooperative Oncology Group (ECOG) 0, no comorbidities Life expectancy likely 2–3 y with systemic therapy only; surgical consolidation may offer potential for cure
Patient goals/values	Desires aggressive treatment with intent to prolong life
Surgical considerations	Patient is an excellent candidate for surgery Surgical appropriateness depends on response of liver metastasis to systemic treatment
Medical oncology considerations	Patient is an appropriate candidate for FOLFOX Limit to 4 preoperative cycles to decrease hepatotoxicity before surgery
Palliative care considerations	No immediate symptomatic needs; consult palliative if requested by patient
Coordinated decision-making	Patient and oncologic team agree on care plan: FOLFOX for 4 cycles, reimaging, and resection of primary tumor and metastasis, depending on response Goal of this treatment plan is cure

interdisciplinary communication, a general knowledge of common systemic cancer therapies may enrich these discussions, particularly as this relates to drug class-specific surgical considerations.

BEYOND PALLIATIVE CHEMOTHERAPY: SYSTEMIC THERAPY RISKS FOR THE SURGICAL PATIENT

Given the increasing number of new systemic treatments and new indications for already-approved agents, it is challenging to remain up to date on the most common and most serious perioperative risks associated with these agents. The continuation of Ms Jones' case explores the challenges surgeons and medical oncologists face when patients with advanced cancer on systemic therapies develop new surgical problems.

Case 1B

Three years after her initial surgery, Ms Jones develops asymptomatic, progressive liver and pelvic metastatic disease. She received FOLFIRI (5-fluorouracil, leucovorin, and irinotecan) and bevacizumab with the intent to control her disease progression. After 6 cycles, she develops a rectovaginal fistula; her liver metastases have resolved. Biopsy of the fistula location reveals metastatic cancer. There are no other sites of active disease. She is still hoping to extend her life "as long as possible." Given her excellent performance status, current disease burden, and response to therapy to date, her team believes she would likely recover from surgery and be able to undergo further cancer-directed therapy. Therefore, her surgery team would like to offer a fistula repair.

Ms Jones inquires about whether a fistula repair is higher risk in light of the treatment she is now receiving.

Question: How should Ms Jones' systemic chemotherapy be managed in the context of a new surgical problem and what are implications of her systemic treatment on operative interventions and recovery?

Several themes emerge from the synthesis of existing pharmacologic and clinical data regarding drug-related impacts on surgical or perioperative risk. The discussion here and the details in **Table 2** highlight the general principles related to infectious, bleeding, clotting, and wound healing risks. When oncologic pharmacists are available, surgical and medical oncologists may benefit from including them in interdisciplinary discussions regarding perioperative management of patients on systemic treatments.

Infectious Risk

Any treatments that cause cytopenias, including many cytotoxic and targeted therapies, may lead to an increased risk of infection and bleeding in the perioperative period.[14] Although growth factors may help to mitigate neutropenia and associated bacterial infection rate,[15] data indicate that some systemic therapies also confer some degree of functional immunosuppression that cannot be corrected with myeloid growth factors.[16]

In addition to leukopenia, some therapies, including cytotoxic chemotherapies, anti-CD20 monoclonal antibodies, corticosteroids, and others increase the risk of opportunistic infections such as *Pneumocystis jirovecii* pneumonia, invasive fungal infections, or JC-virus associated progressive multifocal leukoencephalopathy,[17] which may increase the morbidity of surgery in patients with cancer, as has been observed in HIV-positive patients with active opportunistic infections.[18]

Table 2
Systemic anticancer medications that impair wound healing in the perioperative period

Drug Class	Agent	General Indications	Potential Wound-related Perioperative Complications	Details/Management/Recommendations
Cytotoxic chemotherapies	Alkylating agents (eg, cyclophosphamide, cisplatin) Antimetabolites (eg, 5-fluourouracil, methotrexate, azathioprine, cytarabine) Antitumor antibiotics (eg, doxorubicin) Antimicrotubule agents (eg, Taxanes, vincristine, vinblastine)	Widely used in the treatment of hematologic and solid tumors	Early animal studies indicated negative effect on wound healing Human studies less definitive Risk of infection if patient is cytopenic	General: When feasible, delay postoperative cytotoxic chemotherapy for several weeks; details related to specific agents provided below, if known.[14] Alkylating agents: May decrease wound tensile strength. Antimetabolites: May decrease wound tensile strength and healing. Antitumor antibiotics: delayed wound healing; Doxorubicin: Preoperatively: Hold for 7 d Postoperatively: Hold 7 d if feasible to lessen macrophage mediated wound healing impairment

| Vascular endothelial growth receptor inhibitors | Bevacizumab Ramucirumab | Bevacizumab: Widely used: mCRC, brain, lung, HCC, ovarian, cervical malignancies Ramucirumab: GI, mCRC, lung, HCC malignancies | Impaired wound healing, GI perforation | Bevacizumab Preoperatively: Hold minimum of 6 wk before elective surgery if feasible. Hold for shorter duration for smaller procedures such as port placement. Postoperatively: Hold at least 28 d postoperatively; hold bevacizumab if any wound healing issues develop after restarting. Ramicirumab: Shorter half-life than bevacizumab. Preoperatively: Hold 28 d before elective surgery. Postoperatively: Hold 2 wk after surgery. Both: After waiting minimum recommended postoperative period, assess for adequate wound healing before reinitiation. |

(continued on next page)

Table 2
(continued)

Drug Class	Agent	General Indications	Potential Wound-related Perioperative Complications	Details/Management/ Recommendations
Multi-kinase inhibitors and other agents with antiangiogenic mechanisms	Regorafenib Sorafenib Sunitinib Pazopanib Axitinib Vandetanib Cabozantinib Lenvatinib Ziv-aflibercept	Regorafenib: mCRC, GIST, HCC Sorafenib: RCC, HCC, thyroid Sunitinib: RCC, GIST, pNET Pazopanib: RCC, STS Axitinib: RCC Vandetanib: thyroid Cabozantinib: thyroid, RCC, HCC Lenvatinib: thyroid Ziv-aflibercept: mCRC	Impaired wound healing, GI perforation	For all agents, preoperative recommendations are made in context of elective surgery; After minimum recommended postoperative period, assess for adequate healing before starting medication. Regorafenib: Preoperatively: Hold 2 wk. Postoperatively: Hold least 2 wk. Sorafenib: Preoperatively: Hold at least 10 d. Postoperatively: Hold at least 2 wk. Sunitinib: Preoperatively: Hold at least 3 wk. Postoperatively: Hold at least 2 wk. Pazopinib: Preoperatively: Discontinue at least 7 d. Postoperatively: Assess wound healing before restarting; do not administer if documented wound dehiscence. Axitinib:

Preoperatively: Hold at least 2 d.

Postoperatively: Hold at least 2 wk.

Vandetanib:

Preoperatively: Hold for at least 1 mo.

Postoperatively: Hold for at least 2 wk.

Cabozantinib:

Preoperatively: Hold at least 3 wk

Postoperatively: Hold at least 2 wk

Lenvatinib:

Preoperatively: Hold at least 1 wk.

Postoperatively: Hold at least 2 wk.

Ziv-aflibercept:

Preoperatively: Hold for at least 4 wk.

Postoperatively: Hold for at least 4 wk; discontinue if wound healing is impaired.

(continued on next page)

Table 2
(continued)

Drug Class	Agent	General Indications	Potential Wound-related Perioperative Complications	Details/Management/Recommendations
Corticosteroids	Glucocorticoids	Intermittent use to prevent chemotherapy-induced nausea/vomiting for postoperative nausea/vomiting Higher doses, often with prolonged tapers, indicated to manage edema from brain tumors or immune-related adverse events associated with immunotherapies	Impaired wound healing, wound infections, poor glucose control	Long term (>30 d) use at higher doses associated with greatest risk of wound infection, impaired healing (Santos et al,[14] 2017). If feasible, taper/stop steroids before surgery and limit doses in postoperative period.

Abbreviations: GI, gastrointestinal; GIST, gastrointestinal stromal tumor; HCC, hepatocellular carcinoma; mCRC, metastatic colorectal cancer; pNET, pancreatic neuroendocrine tumor; RCC, renal cell carcinoma.

Data From refs [14, 21, 24, 29–39]

Bleeding and Clotting Complications

In addition to infectious risks from cytopenias, therapies resulting in myelosuppression may also elevate the risk for clinically significant bleeding. Although transfusions present a logical solution to thrombocytopenia, certain targeted therapies such as Bruton's tyrosine kinase inhibitors increase the risk for hemorrhage, irrespective of platelet count.[19]

In addition to increasing the risk of bleeding, specific systemic treatments, such as cisplatin, immunomodulators like thalidomide, corticosteroids, antiangiogenic medications, and hormonal agents such as tamoxifen are associated with elevated risk of venous thromboembolic events (VTE)[20–22] above and beyond the inherent VTE risk from malignancy itself. In the case of tamoxifen, guidelines recommend holding the drug for at least 3 weeks before elective surgery and restarting it when the postoperative VTE risk is decreased.[23] In most situations, patients undergoing cancer surgeries should receive pharmacologic VTE prophylaxis beginning preoperatively and continuing for 7 to 10 days postoperatively or longer if recommended owing to the VTE risk associated with the operation.[24]

Wound Healing

Effective wound healing requires a coordinated series of cellular changes, and the cells and growth factors that facilitate the inflammatory, proliferative and maturation phases of wound healing can be impacted by a variety of systemic cancer therapies.[14] **Table 2** provides general guidance on systemic anti-cancer agents that impact perioperative wound healing, including available evidence regarding recommended length of perioperative abstinence from systemic treatments.

- Cytotoxic chemotherapies

    Cytotoxic chemotherapy works by disrupting cellular division in cancer cells. In addition to tumor cells, bone marrow and gastrointestinal tract cells are impacted, as are cells that mediate the body's response to inflammation and facilitate healing. Although animal models suggest exposure to various cytotoxic chemotherapies may impair wound healing, the direct evidence in human studies is limited.[14] However, most oncologists and surgeons err on the side of caution when considering surgical interventions in patients who have recently received cytotoxic agents.

- Antiangiogenic agents

    Bevacizumab is the prototypical vascular endothelial growth factor–targeted therapy causing wound healing issues in the perioperative period. It is also associated with gastrointestinal perforations, bleeding, and arterial thrombotic events.[21,22] Owing to its long half-life, it is recommended that bevacizumab be held at least 6 weeks before elective surgeries, and at least 28 days postoperatively or until the surgical wound has healed.[25] Many multikinase inhibitors that target the vascular endothelial growth factor pathway have shorter half-lives, and evidence is accruing regarding specific length of preoperative and postoperative is abstinence required in the setting of surgery (**Table 2**).

- Immunotherapeutic agents

    In the last 10 years, several immune checkpoint inhibitors have been approved and indications are expanding. To date, there are no substantial data that immune checkpoint inhibitors are linked directly to significant perioperative complications, such as wound healing complications.[26,27] However, they are associated with numerous immune-related adverse events, including endocrinopathies and pneumonitis, which could impact a patient's perioperative recovery.[27] If immune-related adverse events are severe, patients often require prolonged course of high dose steroids,[28] placing them at risk for wound healing complications if surgery is required before or during this period (discussed elsewhere in this article).

- Corticosteroids

  Patients with advanced cancer receive corticosteroids for many indications, including prophylaxis or the management of nausea and vomiting, as a part of chemotherapy regimens, and as a treatment for cancer- or treatment-associated symptoms. Longer exposure and higher doses of corticosteroids increase the risk for postoperative wound complications. Furthermore, patients with diabetes taking steroids may have poorly controlled blood glucose levels, contributing to wound complications.[29]

Although not exhaustive, understanding basic perioperative risks associated with systemic treatments frequently prescribed to patients with advanced cancer can help guide surgical planning for patients. Interdisciplinary discussion regarding patient-specific recommendations remains the gold standard and will account for individual patient- and disease-related factors that could impact the timing and/or length of perioperative systemic treatment holiday. **Table 3** presents the decision-making process for case 1B.

Table 3	
Case 1B: Ms Jones has received palliative chemotherapy and now needs surgery	
Prognostic considerations	ECOG 0–1 Limited burden of metastatic disease at time of fistula development Estimated life expectancy of multiple months to several years
Patient goals/values	Continues to desire disease-directed treatment with intent to prolong life; new grandchild was born recently Living with fistula is distressing; she would like it repaired
Surgical considerations	Fistula repair feasible Surgical intent is noncurative Goal: to improve patient quality of life and function
Medical oncology considerations	Current therapy: FOLFIRI and bevacizumab given with noncurative intent; Perioperative management: Hold bevacizumab given anticipated surgery; minimum 6–8 wk before surgery; and 4 wk postoperatively Future therapy: Further systemic treatment is feasible; numerous options available Wound healing postoperatively and restaging will guide decisions on timing of postoperative systemic therapy Ms Jones is at risk for progressive disease in perioperative period; systemic therapy will be held for at least 10 weeks
Palliative care considerations	Patient and oncologists have disease directed plan Ms Jones is distressed by fistula, recurrent disease; offer palliative care consult
Coordinated decision-making:	Surgical plan discussed; patient aware and accepting of required systemic treatment holiday and risk for disease progression; patient seeks fistula repair for improved quality of life Surgery scheduled in 6 wk

Case 1B Conclusion

FOLFIRI and bevacizumab are held, and Ms Jones undergoes an abdominoperineal resection with end colostomy, posterior vaginectomy, and gracilis flap reconstruction, complicated by partial flap failure requiring multiple debridements. The palliative care team was consulted to help manage complex somatic and neuropathic postoperative pain. Ultimately, she resumed cytotoxic chemotherapy and completed 6 months of FOLFIRI before her functional status declined from ECOG 0 to ECOG 2. She has no measurable metastatic disease, so a treatment break was recommended.

WHEN SYSTEMIC THERAPY AND SURGICAL INTERVENTION ARE NO LONGER APPROPRIATE

Medical decision-making regarding advance cancer treatment, systemic cancer therapies, and surgical intervention is often complex. It requires the integration of information from many team members and must take into account patient goals and values. Collaborative decision-making is especially critical in the setting of urgent or emergent surgical problems that arise when patients are near the end of life. Structured discussions using the same framework can ensure appropriate decision-making and care planning, as illustrated in **Table 4**.

Case 1C

After 6 months off systemic therapies, Ms Jones' carcinoembryonic antigen increases and peritoneal carcinomatosis is identified on imaging. Tumor pathology revealed microsatellite instability and her oncologist suggests a trial of immunotherapy given her debility after her last surgery and chemotherapy. She received 7 cycles of

Table 4	
Case 1C: Ms Jones experiences progressive cancer with bowel obstruction while on third-line systemic therapy	
Prognostic considerations	ECOG 2–3, needing increasing assistance Worsening burden of metastatic disease Estimated life expectancy in the range of weeks to months
Patient goals/values:	Quality of life is poor with intractable nausea and vomiting requiring a nasogastric tube Ms Jones does not wish to die in the hospital
Surgical considerations	Imaging: Peritoneal metastatic deposits causing multiple transition points in the small bowel Venting gastrostomy feasible despite peritoneal disease; offers freedom from the nasogastric tube
Medical oncology considerations	Recent immunotherapy exposure unlikely to impact surgical recovery Progressive cancer on third-line systemic treatment, poor performance status suggests limited benefit to additional systemic treatments
Palliative care considerations	Convene family meeting and contextualize offer for venting gastrostomy in light of patient's stated goals Plan to avoid intensive care unit admission and transition to comfort-focused care acutely if she decompensates in the postoperative period
Coordinated decision-making	Plans are made to pursue venting gastrostomy with a transition to home hospice after the immediate postoperative period

pembrolizumab monotherapy and is then admitted for intractable nausea and vomiting attributed to a malignant small bowel obstruction. Surgical oncology is consulted regarding operative management.

Question: Before making treatment plans for Ms Jones, what clinical and prognostic considerations should be examined by her team?

Case 1C Conclusion

After the gastrostomy procedure Ms Jones has home hospice care arranged. She lives 3 weeks and does not require rehospitalization or transfer to an inpatient hospice facility.

In some instances, the mechanism of action or side effects of systemic cancer therapy may not influence medical decision-making. Rather, decisions are made based on the prognostic implications of available data, including poor ECOG performance status limiting future systemic treatment options, poor response to current palliative systemic therapy, and low likelihood of functional recovery from major surgery. Only through use of a structured communication framework can the medical and surgical team be certain to provide optimal whole person care.

SUMMARY

The management of advanced cancer has undergone a dramatic evolution in recent years. "Palliative chemotherapy" does not adequately describe the abundance of new systemic therapies for advanced cancer and the variety of clinical scenarios in which patients may be offered them. The future of oncology care will require collaborative communication between the surgical and medical oncology team throughout the patient's journey with advanced cancer. Although general pharmacologic principles can provide guidance regarding the perioperative risks of systemic therapies, proactive, direct, interdisciplinary communication will always serve as the foundation of high quality cancer care for patients with advanced malignancies.

CLINICS CARE POINTS

- *Lexical gap:* Palliative chemotherapy is a term that lacks a standard definition. When surgical oncologists care for patients receiving "palliative chemotherapy" in the perioperative period, they should explore:
  - The type of medication being offered;
  - The intent of the systemic therapy (eg, life prolongation, symptom control); and
  - The potential impact of the medication on surgical outcomes.
- *Pharmacology:* Systemic anti-cancer therapies may have perioperative risks such as infection, thromboembolism, and impaired wound healing.
- *Perioperative risk mitigation:* Surgeons should collaborate with medical oncologists and oncology pharmacists to mitigate perioperative risk for patients with advanced cancer receiving perioperative systemic therapies.
- *Values-congruent patient care requires communication:* Structured communication with multidisciplinary team members regarding treatment and disease-related prognosis, treatment intent, and treatment planning can help guide values-based goals of care decisions in the perioperative period.
- *Integrate palliative care early for patients with advanced cancer:* Consider a palliative care consultation when:
  - The patient or family requests palliative care support;
  - Proposed interventions such as surgery and/or systemic therapy carry significant risk;

- ○ Patients have significant symptom burden from their cancer or cancer treatment; and
- ○ Teams require assistance clarifying a patient's goals and values.

DISCLOSURE

E. Wulff-Burchfield: Consulting or advisory role, Exelixis, Astellas; Family member with stock ownership, Immunomedics and Nektar. L. Spoozak: Travel funding, Intuitive Surgical; E. Finlay, MD: Stock ownership, Merck.

REFERENCES

1. Roeland EaTL. Palliative chemotherapy: oxymoron or misunderstanding? BMC Palliat Care 2016;15:33.
2. Neugut AI, Prigerson HG. Curative, life-extending, and palliative chemotherapy: new outcomes need new names. Oncologist 2017;22:883–5.
3. Weissman D. Fast Fact #14: palliative chemotherapy. Fast Fact 2015. Available at: https://www.mypcnow.org/fast-fact/palliative-chemotherapy/. Accessed September 26, 2020.
4. Smith A. "Palliative chemotherapy" - a term that should be laid to rest. In. GeriPal: A Geriatrics and Palliative Care Blog. Available at: https://www.geripal.org/2014/05/palliative-chemotherapy-term-that.html. Accessed September 26, 2020.
5. Burris HA 3rd, Moore MJ, Andersen J, et al. Improvements in survival and clinical benefit with gemcitabine as first-line therapy for patients with advanced pancreas cancer: a randomized trial. J Clin Oncol 1997;15(6):2403–13.
6. Weeks JCCP, Cronin A, Finkelman MD, et al. Patients' expectations about effects of chemotherapy for advanced cancer. N Engl J Med 2012;367(17):1616–25.
7. Ferrell BR, Temel JS, Temin S, et al. Integration of palliative care into standard oncology care: American Society of Clinical Oncology clinical practice guideline update. J Clin Oncol 2017;35(1):96–112.
8. Bakitas MA, Tosteson TD, Li Z, et al. Early versus delayed initiation of concurrent palliative oncology care: patient outcomes in the ENABLE III randomized controlled trial. J Clin Oncol 2015;33(13):1438–45.
9. Zimmermann C, Swami N, Krzyzanowska M, et al. Early palliative care for patients with advanced cancer: a cluster-randomised controlled trial. Lancet 2014; 383(9930):1721–30.
10. Ferrell B, Sun V, Hurria A, et al. Interdisciplinary Palliative Care for Patients With Lung Cancer. J Pain Symptom Manage 2015;50(6):758–67.
11. Temel JS, Greer JA, Muzikansky A, et al. Early palliative care for patients with metastatic non-small-cell lung cancer. N Engl J Med 2010;363(8):733–42.
12. Dictionary OE. "chemotherapy, n.". 2020. Available at: https://www.oed.com/view/Entry/31284?redirectedFrom=chemotherapy. Accessed September 07, 2020.
13. Schwarze ML, Kehler JM, Campbell TC. Navigating high risk procedures with more than just a street map. J Palliat Med 2013;16(10):1169–71.
14. Santos DA, Alseidi A, Shannon VR, et al. Management of surgical challenges in actively treated cancer patients. Curr Probl Surg 2017;54(12):612–54.
15. Kuderer NM, Dale DC, Crawford J, et al. Impact of primary prophylaxis with granulocyte colony-stimulating factor on febrile neutropenia and mortality in adult cancer patients receiving chemotherapy: a systematic review. J Clin Oncol 2007; 25(21):3158–67.

16. Verma R, Foster RE, Horgan K, et al. Lymphocyte depletion and repopulation after chemotherapy for primary breast cancer. Breast Cancer Res 2016;18(1):10.

17. Carson KR, Evens AM, Richey EA, et al. Progressive multifocal leukoencephalopathy after rituximab therapy in HIV-negative patients: a report of 57 cases from the Research on Adverse Drug Events and Reports project. Blood 2009; 113(20):4834–40.

18. King JT Jr, Perkal MF, Rosenthal RA, et al. Thirty-day postoperative mortality among individuals with HIV infection receiving antiretroviral therapy and procedure-matched, uninfected comparators. JAMA Surg 2015;150(4):343–51.

19. Shatzel JJ, Olson SR, Tao DL, et al. Ibrutinib-associated bleeding: pathogenesis, management and risk reduction strategies. J Thromb Haemost 2017;15(5): 835–47.

20. Oppelt P, Betbadal A, Nayak L. Approach to chemotherapy-associated thrombosis. Vasc Med 2015;20(2):153–61.

21. Bailey CE, Parikh AA. Assessment of the risk of antiangiogenic agents before and after surgery. Cancer Treat Rev 2018;68:38–46.

22. Bose D, Meric-Bernstam F, Hofstetter W, et al. Vascular endothelial growth factor targeted therapy in the perioperative setting: implications for patient care. Lancet Oncol 2010;11(4):373–82.

23. Hussain T, Kneeshaw PJ. Stopping tamoxifen peri-operatively for VTE risk reduction: a proposed management algorithm. Int J Surg 2012;10(6):313–6.

24. Key NS, Khorana AA, Kuderer NM, et al. Venous Thromboembolism Prophylaxis and Treatment in Patients With Cancer: ASCO clinical practice guideline update. J Clin Oncol 2020;38(5):496–520.

25. AVASTIN (bevacizumab) [package insert]. Available at: https://www.gene.com/download/pdf/avastin_prescribing.pdf. Accessed August 29, 2020.

26. Sun J, Kirichenko DA, Chung JL, et al. Perioperative Outcomes of Melanoma Patients Undergoing Surgery After Receiving Immunotherapy or Targeted Therapy. World J Surg 2020;44(4):1283–93.

27. Santos DA, Alseidi A, Shannon VR, et al. Management of surgical challenges in actively treated cancer patients. Curr Probl Surg 2017;54(12):612–54.

28. Brahmer JR, Lacchetti C, Schneider BJ, et al. Management of immune-related adverse events in patients treated with immune checkpoint inhibitor therapy: American Society of Clinical Oncology clinical practice guideline. J Clin Oncol 2018;36(17):1714–68.

29. Mathiesen O, Wetterslev J, Kontinen VK, et al. Adverse effects of perioperative paracetamol, NSAIDs, glucocorticoids, gabapentinoids and their combinations: a topical review. Acta Anaesthesiol Scand 2014;58(10):1182–98.

30. CYRAMZA (ramucirumab) [package insert]. 2020. Available at: https://www.accessdata.fda.gov/drugsatfda_docs/label/2014/125477lbl.pdf.   Accessed August 29, 2020.

31. STIVARGA (regorafenib) [package insert]. 2020; STIVARGA (regorafenib) package insert. 2020. Available at: http://labeling.bayerhealthcare.com/html/products/pi/Stivarga_PI.pdf. Accessed August 29, 2020.

32. NEXAVAR (sorafenib) [package insert]. 2020. Available at: http://labeling.bayerhealthcare.com/html/products/pi/Nexavar_PI.pdf. Accessed August 29, 2020.

33. CABOMETYX (cabozantinib) [package insert]. 2020. Available at: https://www.cabometyxhcp.com/downloads/CABOMETYXUSPI.pdf. Accessed August 29, 2020.

34. SUTENT (sunitinib malate) [Package Insert]. 2020. Available at: http://labeling. pfizer.com/showlabeling.aspx?id=607. Accessed August 29, 2020.
35. VOTRIENT (pazopanib) [package insert]. 2020. Available at: https://www. novartis.us/sites/www.novartis.us/files/votrient.pdf. Accessed August 29, 2020.
36. INLYTA (axitinib) [package insert]. 2020. Available at: http://labeling.pfizer.com/ ShowLabeling.aspx?id=759. Accessed August 29, 2020.
37. CAPRELSA (vandetanib) [package insert]. 2020. Available at: https://www. caprelsa.com/files/caprelsa-pi.pdf. Accessed August 29, 2020.
38. LENVIMA (lenvatinib) [package insert]. 2020. Available at: http://www.lenvima. com/pdfs/prescribing-information.pdf. Accessed August 29, 2020.
39. ZALTRAP (ziv-aflibercept) [package insert]. 2020. Available at: http://products. sanofi.us/Zaltrap/Zaltrap.html. Accessed August 29, 2020.

Palliative Radiotherapy for Advanced Cancers

Indications and Outcomes

Graeme R. Williams, MD, MBA[a,b,*,1],
Shwetha H. Manjunath, MD[a,1], Anish A. Butala, MD[a],
Joshua A. Jones, MD, MA[a]

KEYWORDS

- Palliative radiotherapy • Palliative care • Supportive oncology • Radiation oncology

KEY POINTS

- Palliative radiotherapy is a safe, versatile, and effective therapy for various symptoms of advanced cancer.
- Indications for palliative radiotherapy are expanding from pure palliation to modifying the natural history of disease.
- A growing body of evidence supports the use of advance radiotherapy techniques in palliative radiotherapy.

INTRODUCTION

More than 40% of patients with metastatic cancer receive palliative radiotherapy (PRT).[1] PRT is an efficient, cost-effective, well-tolerated, and noninvasive treatment modality that can achieve rapid, durable symptom relief even for patients with poor prognosis.[2] Contemporary paradigms suggest a broader role for radiotherapy (RT) among patients with metastatic disease. Assessment of such patients requires recognition of symptoms and indications that may benefit from PRT. This review (1) defines the role of PRT as it relates to goals of care (GOC), (2) reviews common indications and evidence supporting PRT, and (3) reviews specific PRT options/considerations for common clinical scenarios.

Funding Statement: N/A.
Conflicts of Interest: The authors have no conflicts of interest to disclose.
[a] Department of Radiation Oncology, Hospital of the University of Pennsylvania, Perelman Center for Advanced Medicine, 3400 Civic Center Boulevard, 2nd Floor West, Philadelphia, PA 19104, USA; [b] Leonard Davis Institute of Healthcare Economics, University of Pennsylvania, Philadelphia, PA, USA
[1] These authors contributed equally to this work.
* Corresponding author. Department of Radiation Oncology, Perelman Center for Advanced Medicine, 3400 Civic Center Boulevard, 2nd Floor West, Philadelphia, PA 19104.
E-mail address: Graeme.williams@pennmedicine.upenn.edu

Surg Oncol Clin N Am 30 (2021) 563–580
https://doi.org/10.1016/j.soc.2021.02.007
1055-3207/21/© 2021 Elsevier Inc. All rights reserved.

PATIENT SELECTION FRAMEWORK AND PROGNOSTICATION

Selecting appropriate PRT for a patient requires a multidisciplinary framework hinging on treatment intent. Historically, this was a binary choice between cure and symptom palliation, with the former typically delivered in 1.8- to 2.0-Gy daily fractions over 5 to 9 weeks. PRT regimens generally use hypofractionation (larger doses per fraction with fewer total fractions), balancing clinical efficacy against toxicity and logistical burden.

With advances in cancer care and the recognition of the oligometastatic state as a unique opportunity for long-term survival or potentially cure, defining treatment intent has become more nuanced. Clinicians now consider modifying disease trajectory and providing durable local tumor control in select patients with longer life expectancies. Treatment intent is influenced by factors such as prognosis, performance status, disease burden, radiosensitivity (**Table 1**),[3-7] alternative therapeutic options, potential toxicities, and patient priorities/values/goals.

Prognosis is notoriously challenging to predict with continual therapeutic advancements; physicians frequently overestimate survival of patients with advanced cancer.[8] Therefore, individualizing PRT courses on the sole basis of patient survival remains difficult. Nonetheless, prognostic models, such as TEACHH (*T*ype of cancer, *E*astern Cooperative Oncology Group performance status, *A*ge, prior palliative *C*hemotherapy, prior *H*ospitalizations, and *H*epatic metastases) and Chow's three variable number of risk factors[9] are valuable tools. Recent work to improve prognostication beyond traditional models for patients with symptomatic bone metastases has led to the creation of the Bone Metastases Ensemble Trees for Survival machine learning model, which uses 27 prognostic covariates to create patient-specific predicted survival curves.[10]

COMMON REASONS FOR CONSULTATION
Pain

Pain affects greater than 60% of patients with advanced cancers[11] caused by metastases, uncontrolled primary disease, or complications from therapy. RT can offer effective palliation of painful malignant lesions by reducing tumor size and modulating pain signaling pathways,[12] offering relief even if tumor response is minimal. Analgesia from PRT is best studied for bone metastases demonstrating response rates of greater than or equal to 60%,[13] but is also effective for other advanced cancers.

Clinicians should ensure medical management is optimized because one-third of patients' symptoms are inadequately controlled at baseline.[14] PRT may help de-escalate pain medications, but patients often benefit from continued use of opioids, adjuvants, and corticosteroids for pain optimization. Additionally, all patients with advanced cancers should be considered for palliative care consultation to ease

Table 1 Radiosensitivity of select histologies	
Radiosensitive	**Radioresistant**
Lymphoma	Sarcoma
Myeloma	Renal cell carcinoma
Seminoma	Melanoma
Breast	Gastrointestinal
Prostate	

Data from Katsoulakis E, Kumar K, Laufer I, Yamada Y. Stereotactic Body Radiotherapy in the Treatment of Spinal Metastases. *Semin Radiat Oncol.* 2017;27(3):209-217.

pain and other physical and psychosocial symptoms known to potentiate physical and mental suffering.

Bleeding

Bleeding affects up to 10% of patients with advanced cancers[15] presenting as hemoptysis, hematemesis, hematochezia, hematuria, menorrhagia, or bleeding from fungating disease, and may require admission for urgent stabilization. Multidisciplinary management is necessary with medication management, systemic therapies, wound care, interventional procedures (surgery or embolization), and PRT all playing a potential role.

For patients stable enough for PRT, radiation can achieve hemostasis via tumor response, small vessel damage, and upregulation of the hemostatic cascade.[16,17] In some cases of advanced but curable disease, RT can temporize and stabilize before pursuing a more definitive treatment course.

Series suggest modest radiation doses can achieve hemostasis in up to 80% of patients, including primaries of the breast,[18] stomach,[19] cervix,[20] rectum,[21] prostate,[22] and skin,[23] among others. Our institution typically uses hypofractionated regimens with total doses 9 to 30 Gy in 3- to 10-Gy fractions with higher doses reserved for patients with good prognosis and few metastases.

Local Control

Local control, often studied in curative settings, is equally important in palliating advanced disease for patients with good prognosis. It is particularly important in the brain, spine, head and neck (H&N), and pelvis,[24] because loss of local control can result in severe morbidity and mortality, and present complicated, costly management challenges.

The most studied indications are metastatic cord compression and brain metastases (BM), but evidence supporting PRT for obstruction involving major airways, digestive/biliary tracts, major vessels, or genitourinary (GU) tract sites also exists. Clinical decision-making depends on harm-benefit assessment and multidisciplinary discussion, with prognosis and GOC informing recommendations.

PALLIATION OF PRIMARY SITES

Considerations for each disease site have led to focused research specific to histology and anatomic location. Herein we review data for managing advanced primary tumors of different sites. A summarized framework with treatment options and references follows in **Table 2**.

Head and Neck

PRT for cancers of the H&N offers a range of options from definitive management over 6 to 7 weeks to hypofractionated schedules, such as 0-7-21 or the Quad Shot regimen (3.7 Gy twice daily for four fractions repeated monthly up to three times). A recent review of treatment options offers the framework included in **Fig. 1**, which incorporates assessment of the patient, burden of disease, prior therapy, multidisciplinary discussion, toxicity risk, and GOC to inform decision-making.[25] This framework can be generalized to many primary sites.

Multiple trials conducted since 1993 have reported response rates ranging from 40% to greater than 80%, with even the shortest regimens (Quad Shot; 0-7-21) having response rates greater than 80%. In definitive treatment of H&N cancers 6 to 7 weeks of curative-intent concurrent chemoradiation can have significant side effects, but most trials in the palliative setting report toxicities in the range of less than or equal

Table 2
Treatment options for palliative radiotherapy of primary sites

Site	Prognosis	Regimen	Fractionation
Multiple	<4 mo		8 Gy/1 fx 20 Gy/5 fx 30 Gy/10 fx Supportive care only/hospice
Head and neck[25]	<4 mo 4–12 mo >12 mo	Quad Shot Porceddu Tata & Christie	14.8 Gy/4 fx BID (up to 3 cycles) 21 Gy/3 fx 30–32 Gy/5–8 fx 40–50 Gy/16 fx 60 Gy/20 fx 70 Gy/35 fx Chemoradiotherapy
Lung/thorax[26]	<4 mo 4–12 mo	Sundstrom	10 Gy/1 fx 17 Gy/2 fx (weekly) 30–40 Gy/10–15 fx 45 Gy/15 fx Chemoradiotherapy Intraluminal HDR brachytherapy
Breast[18]	All appropriate for short- or long-term prognosis patients	Rutgers UK FAST and Dragun UK FAST-Forward UK START Whelan	36.63 Gy/11 fx 30 Gy/5 fx 28.5 Gy/5 fx 27 Gy/5 fx 26 Gy/5 fx 40.05 Gy/15 fx 42.56 Gy/16 fx
Gastrointestinal (esophagus, stomach, colorectal cancers)	<4 mo 4–12 mo >12 mo	TROG 03.01	24 Gy/3 fx 30–35 Gy/10–15 fx 35 Gy/15 fx 50 Gy/25 fx Chemoradiotherapy Intraluminal HDR brachytherapy
Gynecologic (endometrial, cervical, vaginal cancers	<4 mo 4–12 mo >12 mo	Quad Shot 0-7-21	14.8 Gy/4 fx BID (up to 3 cycles) 7–8 Gy/1 fx on Day 0, 7, and 21 as needed 10 Gy/1 fx monthly up to 3 times 30 Gy/10 fx 50 Gy/20 fx HDR brachytherapy
Genitourinary (bladder cancer, prostate cancer)	<4 mo 4–12 mo >12 mo	Quad Shot MRC BA09	14.8 Gy/4 fx BID (up to 3 cycles) 21 Gy/3 fx delivered QOD 30–35 Gy/10 fx

(continued on next page)

Table 2
(*continued*)

Site	Prognosis	Regimen	Fractionation
			50–60 Gy/20–30 fx
			HDR brachytherapy
Extremity/bone	<4 mo		30 Gy/5 fx
	4–12 mo		30–40 Gy/10–15 fx
	>12 mo		50 Gy/25 fx
			66 Gy/33 fx
Skin	<4 mo	Princess Margaret	24 Gy/3 fx over 3 wk
	4–12 mo		30–35 Gy/5 fx over
	>12 mo		3 wk
			50 Gy/20 fx
			55 Gy/20 fx
			50–70 Gy/25–35 fx

Abbreviations: BID, twice daily fractionation; fx, fractions; HDR, high dose rate.

Data from Grewal AS, Jones J, Lin A. Palliative Radiation Therapy for Head and Neck Cancers. *Int J Radiat Oncol Biol Phys.* 2019;105(2):254-266.; Rodrigues G, Videtic GM, Sur R, et al. Palliative thoracic radiotherapy in lung cancer: An American Society for Radiation Oncology evidence-based clinical practice guideline. *Pract Radiat Oncol.* 2011;1(2):60-71; and Grewal AS, Freedman GM, Jones JA, Taunk NK. Hypofractionated radiation therapy for durable palliative treatment of bleeding, fungating breast cancers. *Pract Radiat Oncol.* 2019;9(2).

to 30% to 40% grade 3, with less than 5% grade 4 and no grade 5 toxicity. Thus, PRT for advanced H&N cancers offers a reasonable probability of palliation at the cost of modest acute toxicity.

Thoracic

Advanced thoracic malignancies and lung metastases cause cough, hemoptysis, hematemesis, chest wall pain, dysphagia, odynophagia, or airway obstruction resulting in respiratory distress and/or postobstructive pneumonia requiring PRT.

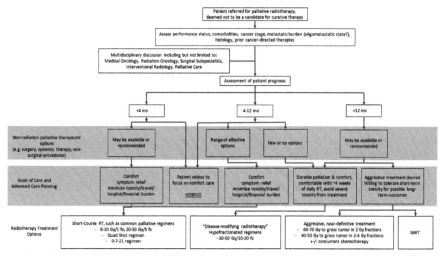

Fig. 1. Palliative RT framework. SBRT, stereotactic body radiotherapy. (*Adapted from* Grewal AS, Jones J, Lin A. Palliative Radiation Therapy for Head and Neck Cancers. Int J Radiat Oncol Biol Phys. 2019;105(2):254-266., with permission.)

PRT studies for non–small cell lung cancer (NSCLC) demonstrate the importance of prognosis for decision-making. Higher dose PRT regimens may improve survival or tumor control at the cost of treatment-related toxicity,[26] but a large systematic review found no survival difference when controlling for performance status.[27] Additionally, patients with stage III disease not amenable for curative-intent therapy should be considered for concurrent hypofractionated chemoradiotherapy if they have adequate performance status and life expectancy.[28] Depending on prognosis, traditional palliative regimens (20 Gy in 5 fractions or 30 Gy in 10 fractions) may be appropriate, whereas patients with longer survival may benefit from dose escalation to 45 to 50 Gy in 2.5- to 3-Gy fractions.

For patients with extensive stage small cell lung cancer, consolidative thoracic RT was shown to improve survival, but subsequent publications note discretion in patient selection is essential.[29] Patients with bulky mediastinal disease are at risk of complications and symptoms from local failure and may benefit from thoracic PRT. A 30 Gy in 10 fractions is well-tolerated in randomized clinical trials (RCTs) and an ideal palliative schedule for small cell lung cancer, but guidelines suggest higher doses may be appropriate for patients expected to have prolonged survival.

Breast

Presentation of advanced breast cancers can range from uncontrolled primary lesions resulting in pain, ulceration, or bleeding to advanced nodal disease of the axilla or low neck. Published PRT series include 30 Gy in 15 fractions[30] or 36.63 Gy in 11 fractions,[18] and slightly higher dose hypofractionated regimens offering low toxicities as would be used in definitive treatment paradigms. The literature notes the value of local control in these patients, because even those with advanced disease can live for many years. Radiobiologically, moderately hypofractionated PRT may offer the best possibility for durable local control.

Gastrointestinal

Advanced gastrointestinal tumors may cause obstruction, compression, pain, or bleeding. In esophageal cancer, dysphagia is relieved by external beam PRT, stent placement, endoscopic ablative treatment, or a combination thereof.

Esophageal stenting offers immediate relief and is recommended for patients with near-total obstruction or limited prognosis. However, tumor overgrowth compromises patency in approximately 12% of patients. Compared with stenting, PRT poses a lower risk of perforation, fistula, or hemorrhage while providing equivalent relief of dysphagia and greater relief of pain.[31] Additionally, PRT post-stenting improves dysphagia-free survival from 3 to 4 months.[32]

Common hypofractionated PRT regimens for dysphagia include 20 Gy in five fractions, 30 Gy in 10 fractions, and 35 Gy in 15 fractions.[33] Brief courses have been shown to be effective for greater than 50% of symptoms without grade 3 or higher toxicity.[34] Palliative chemotherapy may be incorporated with local PRT, although randomized evidence suggests similar dysphagia relief with increased toxicity.[33] Intraluminal brachytherapy (BT) also has high response rates (87%),[35] but if incorrectly performed can cause catastrophic consequences.

Biliary obstruction from cholangiocarcinoma often requires upfront stenting and can be followed by palliative external beam RT or intraluminal BT. In unresectable gastric cancer, PRT courses of 1 to 10 fractions are well tolerated and can alleviate bleeding, pyloric obstruction, and pain with response rates of 70% to 75% lasting 3 to 7 months.[36,37] Patients with rectal cancer not undergoing palliative resection can benefit from aggressive or short-course PRT (ie, 45–60 Gy in 25–30 fractions or 25–30 Gy in 5–6 fractions). Both regimens provide comparable rates of pain relief, tumor control, and hemostasis (50%–80%) with median symptom recurrence at 5 months.[38] Concurrent chemoradiotherapy with fluorouracil is best for patients with good performance status and prognosis greater than 6 months.

Genitourinary

Advanced cancers arising from the GU system can cause hematuria, pain, recurrent urinary tract infections, urinary frequency, dysuria, erectile dysfunction, urinary retention or obstruction, hydronephrosis, or bowel obstruction. Hormonal therapy for prostate cancer and chemoimmunotherapy for bladder cancer are fundamental to the treatment and prevention of local symptoms. PRT can significantly lower rates of bleeding, pain, and obstruction.

Randomized evidence has demonstrated equivalent efficacy and toxicity between 21 Gy in three fractions and 35 Gy in 10 fractions for bladder cancer.[39] As seen in other disease sites, higher dose regimens did not translate into better palliation. In fact, prolonged PRT courses can inadvertently increase toxicity without benefit.[40] Patients with castration-resistant prostate cancer can similarly achieve palliation when treated to a total dose of 45 to 60 Gy in 2.0 to 2.5 Gy per fraction.[41]

Gynecologic

Advanced gynecologic tumors may cause vaginal bleeding, pain, dyspareunia, lymphedema, and compression of adjacent organs (gastrointestinal and GU). Hypofractionated PRT or BT can offer rapid hemostasis in locally advanced or recurrent cervical, endometrial, and vaginal cancers.[42]

A seminal study established the Quad Shot (3.7 Gy twice daily for four fractions repeated monthly up to three times) as a safe schedule highly effective for pain, bleeding, and obstipation.[43] The three-fraction course, 0-7-21, has also demonstrated excellent bleeding and pain control with low toxicity.[44] As in H&N cancers, these versatile regimens allow for evaluation of response and toxicity to guide decisions on total dose.

Because long- (ie, >5 fractions) and short-course PRT offer equal hemostasis and durability, short courses are preferable to reduce treatment burden and financial toxicity. These considerations are especially important in light of racial disparities in presentation, treatment, and outcomes between black and white women with endometrial and cervical cancer.[45,46]

Palliative options for locoregional recurrence from gynecologic malignancies depend on prior RT. For women without prior pelvic RT, curative intent external beam RT plus intracavitary/interstitial BT is recommended. For women with prior pelvic RT, reirradiation with external beam RT or incavitary/interstitial BT may be performed to small tumor volumes minimizing overlap. Alternatively, patients with prior incavitary/interstitial BT only may receive salvage surgery with intraoperative RT.[47] Pelvic exenteration is reserved as a last resort because of its significant morbidity.

Extremity, Bone, and Skin

By alleviating pain, bleeding, ulceration, lymphedema, and neurologic symptoms, PRT improves the quality of life in patients with skin cancers and sarcomas. Management of skin malignancies requires consideration of cosmetic and psychosocial outcomes in conjunction with tumor control. Fractionation schemes of 24 to 35 Gy in three to six fractions for basal and squamous cell carcinomas balance dose-related toxicity with response. For melanoma, larger fraction sizes (ie, $\geq$4 Gy per fraction to a total dose of >30 Gy) improve palliation and local control given its radioresistance.[23,48]

Advanced sarcomas often require systemic therapy with PRT delivered for local symptomatic relief. PRT is a recommended treatment option for palliation by the European Society of Medical Oncology[49] despite lack of robust data to guide optimal dose-fractionation. In a retrospective study of sarcomas treated with varying regimens (eg, 8 Gy in 1 fraction, 20 Gy in 5 fractions, 30–40 Gy in 10–15 fractions) PRT improved symptoms in 67% of patients.[50] Despite concerns over treatment-related morbidity, hypofractionated PRT and stereotactic body RT (SBRT) are promising choices for advanced sarcomas. Patients treated with 30 Gy in five fractions followed by immediate or delayed resection experience acceptable wound complications and reduction in treatment package time relative to conventional RT (50 Gy in 25 fractions) followed by delayed surgery.[51] With careful treatment planning, SBRT in recurrent sarcoma provides safe and effective local control and pain relief.[52]

PALLIATION OF METASTATIC SITES
Brain Metastases

BM may develop in up to 30% of patients with solid tumors[53] requiring special consideration given the potential for morbidity and neurologic death from uncontrolled intracranial progression. Treatment options include surgery, systemic therapy, and RT, alone or in combination.

Given the prognostic implications of BM, various systems have been developed to predict survival, including some specific for melanoma, NSCLC, and breast primaries.[54,55]

Early studies demonstrated survival benefit for surgery for solitary BM and improved local and/or whole brain control with the addition of RT (stereotactic radiosurgery [SRS] or whole-brain RT [WBRT]) postoperatively.[5,56] Surgery is preferred for rapid reversal of large and/or symptomatic BM and diagnosis for patients presenting with new metastatic disease.

Historically the role of systemic therapy for BM was limited by modest central nervous system penetration. Improved response rates from novel targeted/immune therapies (**Table 3**) raise the possibility of initiating systemic therapy early while periodically re-evaluating response.

RT has a well-defined role in the multidisciplinary management of BM. RT following surgery improves local and/or intracranial control and can prolong survival in patients

Table 3
Brain metastases systemic therapy response rates

Systemic Therapy (Target)	Response Rates (%)
Tyrosine kinase inhibitors (TKI)	
Gefitinib, erlotinib, afatinib (EGFR)	35–88
Osimertinib (EGFR)[73]	54–91
Ceritinib, alectinib, brigatinib (ALK)	35–68
Dabrafenib/vemurafenib (BRAF) ± trametinib (MEK)	18–90
Lapatinib (Her2) + capecitabine	6–66
Immunotherapy	
Pembrolizumab (PD-1)	26–33
Ipilimumab/nivolumab (CTLA4/PD-1)	6–55

Data from Han RH, Dunn GP, Chheda MG, Kim AH. The impact of systemic precision medicine and immunotherapy treatments on brain metastases. Oncotarget. 2019;10(62):6739-6753.

with limited disease. Nonsurgical series focus on the appropriate use of WBRT and SRS (alone or in combination) for management of BM. In general, a tradeoff exists between improved intracranial control of occult microscopic disease with WBRT and neurocognitive decline. Most evidence supports the use of SRS in patients with three or less BM with series demonstrating similar survival between approaches.[57,58] Emerging research examines SRS for more lesions, with older series suggesting total volume of disease treated rather than absolute number is an important predictor of survival.[59,60]

Additionally, although classic WBRT treatment fields are delivered with lateral opposed beams, newer techniques designed to spare the hippocampus from dose (hippocampal avoidance WBRT) have been explored to reduce neurocognitive decline. NRG CC001 was a phase III clinical trial that randomized 518 patients with nonhippocampal BM to standard WBRT with memantine or hippocampal avoidance WBRT with memantine (**Fig. 2**).[61] At 8 months, risk of cognitive failure (executive function, learning, memory) was significantly lower with hippocampal avoidance WBRT without overall survival (OS) differences. For many, this trial has established a new standard of care for patients without metastases in the hippocampal region.

Finally, a contemporary trial examining WBRT versus best supportive care in patients with BM from NSCLC showed no difference in survival and similar quality of life between treatment arms,[62] questioning the role of RT for patients with advanced NSCLC, BM, and short prognosis.

Bone Metastases

Solid tumors commonly metastasize to bone causing pain, pathologic fracture, or compression of nerve roots or the spinal cord. When incorporated into a multidisciplinary plan (eg, pain medication, systemic therapy, bone-modifying agents, surgical

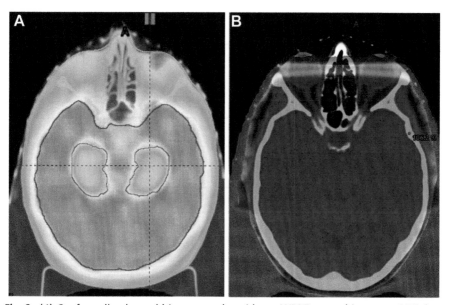

Fig. 2. (*A*) Conformally planned hippocampal avoidance WBRT spares hippocampi RT dose for patients without metastasis involving these regions. (*B*) Standard WBRT uses opposed lateral beams to treat the entire brain uniformly.

stabilization as needed), PRT is highly efficacious and well tolerated. In fact, 60% to 80% of patients experience partial pain relief and 30% to 50% experience complete pain relief within 3 to 4 weeks of starting PRT.[13]

In uncomplicated bone metastases (eg, lesions without a soft tissue component, impending fracture risk, spinal cord/nerve compression, or receipt of prior RT), pain control from single fraction RT is equivalent to longer regimens (ie, $\geq$5 fractions). Although retreatment rates are higher for single versus multifraction PRT, a single 8-Gy fraction is the preferred option for patients with poor prognosis.

However, multifraction PRT is appropriate for lesions following surgical fixation, with associated neuropathic pain, or with associated large soft tissue mass when local control is a secondary goal. If pain from an irradiated bone metastasis recurs or persists, repeat PRT can achieve 50% response rates.[63]

Spinal Cord Compression

Bone metastases of the vertebral column can result in spinal cord compression, which affects 2.5% to 5% of patients with cancer.[64] Cord compression can result in pain, spinal instability, and neurologic sequelae including paralysis, and multidisciplinary management may include neurosurgery, medical oncology, radiation oncology, orthopedics, or interventional radiology.

Medical management should include glucocorticoids to reduce edema contributing to symptoms, aggressive pain control, and consideration of systemic therapies. The NOMS (neurologic, oncologic, mechanical, systemic) Framework (**Table 4**) is used to create an appropriate multidisciplinary plan.

Postoperative radiation treatment is typically delivered over 2 weeks (30 Gy in 10 fractions), whereas patients receiving treatment without prior surgery may be given treatment over 1, 5, or 10 fractions.[65,66] For patients with radioresistant histology or recurrent disease that previously had conventional RT, advanced treatment with SBRT may be considered.

Table 4		
Cord compression (NOMS) framework		
NOMS Framework Component	**Clinical Considerations**	**Treatment Options**
Neurologic	Cord compression severity, presence of myelopathy	Radiosensitive and/or low-grade: treat with conventional RT alone
Oncologic	Radiosensitive vs radioresistant histology	Radioresistant and high-grade: separation surgery followed by SBRT
Mechanical	Stable vs unstable spine	Unstable spine must always be managed before oncologic management, can be surgical or minimally invasive approach, consider RT approach following stabilization
Systemic	Metastatic burden, life expectancy	For patients with short life expectancy, conventional RT only may be appropriate

Data from Katsoulakis E, Kumar K, Laufer I, Yamada Y. Stereotactic Body Radiotherapy in the Treatment of Spinal Metastases. Semin Radiat Oncol. 2017;27(3):209-217.

THE FUTURE OF PALLIATIVE RADIOTHERAPY
Disease-Modifying Radiotherapy: a New Category of Noncurative Intent

Historically, PRT was reserved for symptomatic disease sites but is now also considered for minimally symptomatic or asymptomatic sites with the goal of providing durable local control and/or modifying the natural history of disease. Recent data have shown patients with oligometastatic disease (<3–5 metastases) may benefit from prolonged survival following early local consolidative therapy (**Table 5**). The SABR-COMET trial demonstrated that in patients with controlled primary tumors and one to five oligometastases, SBRT to active disease sites improves OS by 22 months.[67] Confirmatory phase III trials are ongoing.

Irradiating the primary tumor alone in patients with low-burden metastases also seems to modify the clinical trajectory of various cancers. In the STAMPEDE trial, men with de novo low-burden metastatic prostate cancer receiving RT to the prostate had a 17% failure-free survival and 8% OS benefit within the first 3 years post-treatment with no increase in grade 3 toxicity.[68] In synchronous oligometastatic NSCLC, although no RCTs support treating the primary in isolation, a metanalysis of 668 patient showed that thoracic RT significantly improved OS.[69] In extensive stage small cell lung cancer in the preimmunotherapy era, palliative-dose RT to residual thoracic disease conferred a 3% to 13% OS benefit at 2 years.[70] Furthermore, the addition of aggressive locoregional radiation in chemoresponsive patients with de novo metastatic nasopharyngeal carcinoma improved survival from 55% to 76%.[71]

Advanced Technologies in Palliative Radiotherapy

Evolving diagnostic imaging, surgical techniques, and novel therapeutics are improving detection and survival for many cancers. Consequently, many patients with advanced disease are heavily pretreated, and radiation oncologists need to consider the use of advanced technologies to optimize tumor control and/or minimize toxicities. Principle among these technologies are intensity-modulated RT (IMRT), SBRT, and particle therapy.

IMRT is an advanced planning technique to generate treatment plans that conform closely to the edges of a target. It has been adopted as standard for definitive treatment of most primary tumors, whereas PRT often relies on simpler planning techniques that permit shorter treatment times and more reproducible patient positioning. However, IMRT may permit superior normal tissue sparing, potentially decreasing side effects, although this has yet to be confirmed in RCTs for many sites.

Another form of IMRT, SBRT precisely delivers "ablative" RT doses in five or fewer fractions to extracranial targets. Well-established for treatment of isolated lung, liver, or spine lesions, SBRT relies on advanced planning, targeting, and patient immobilization to deliver high doses and may be preferable in cases of limited metastatic disease, radioresistant histologies, or reirradiation.

Finally, although conventional RT relies on photons or electrons to deliver dose to target tissues, particle therapy uses heavy particles (protons, neutrons, or carbon ions) to treat tumor. In the United States proton therapy is the most widely available, with neutrons available at only a handful of sites, and carbon ions only in Europe and Asia. The theoretic advantage of particle therapy results from the physical nature of the beam delivery, whereby dose is deposited as the particle loses momentum, and no dose is delivered distal to the end of the particle's range. This phenomenon results in sparing of tissues distal to the target, with some uncertainty (**Fig. 3**). Use of proton therapy for palliation has been published for H&N cancers,[72] but is otherwise limited. Appropriate clinical use of particle therapy requires experience, consideration of clinical risks/benefits, and potential financial implications of treatment.

Table 5
Summary of evidence supporting aggressive treatment of oligometastatic disease

Disease Site	Trial	Population	Intervention	Outcome
Prostate	STAMPEDE-RT[68]	Patients with metastatic hormone-sensitive prostate cancer (n = 2061)	SOC + prostate RT (55 Gy/20 fx or 36 Gy/6 fx) vs SOC	No OS benefit to the addition of prostate RT in unselect patients Improved OS from 73% vs 81% at 3 y in low-burden metastatic burden disease (as per CHAARTED trial)
Prostate	ORIOLE[74]	Patients with recurrent hormone-sensitive prostate cancer with 1–3 metastases (received no ADT within 6 mo of enrollment or 3 or more y total) (n = 54)	SBRT (19.5–48 Gy/3–5 fx) vs observation	mPFS not reached vs 5.8 mo (SBRT vs observation)
NSCLC	Gomez et al[75]	Patients with 3 or fewer metastatic lesions without progression after first-line systemic therapy (n = 99)	LCT (CRT/RT or surgery) ± maintenance therapy vs maintenance therapy alone or observation (no LCT)	Local progression 52% with LCT vs 70.8% in no LCT mPFS 11.9 mo vs 3.9 mo, 1 y PFS 48% vs 20% (consolidative vs maintenance)
NSCLC	Iyengar et al[76]	Oligometastatic patients with primary disease plus up to 5 metastases (n = 29)	SBRT + maintenance therapy vs maintenance therapy alone	PFS 9.7 mo vs 3.5 mo (SBRT + maintenance therapy vs maintenance therapy alone)
Nasopharynx	You et al[71]	Chemosensitive patients with de novo metastatic nasopharynx cancer (n = 126)	Chemotherapy + RT vs chemotherapy alone	OS 76.4% vs 54.5% at 2 y (chemotherapy + RT vs chemotherapy alone) PFS 35.0% vs 3.6% at 2 y
Mixed	SABR-COMET[77]	Patients with controlled primary Tumor and 1–5 metastatic lesions (93%–94% with 1–3 metastases) (n = 49)	SOC palliative treatment vs SOC + SBRT	mOS 41 mo vs 28 mo, mPFS 12.0 mo vs 6.0 mo (SOC vs SOC + SBRT)
Mixed	SABR-COMET-10[78]	Patients with controlled primary Tumor and 4–10 metastatic lesions (n = 159)	SOC palliative Treatment vs SOC + SBRT	Accruing, primary end point OS and secondary end points include PFS, time to new metastases, quality of life, and toxicity

Abbreviations: ADT, androgen-deprivation therapy; CRT, chemoradiotherapy; LCT, local consolidative therapy; mPFS, median progression-free survival; SOC, standard of care.

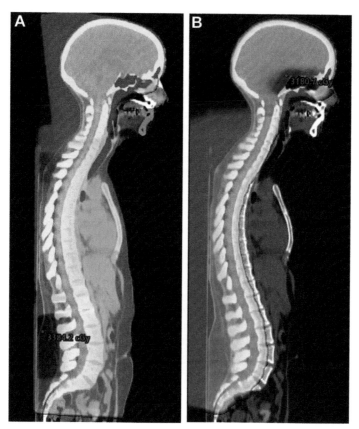

Fig. 3. Craniospinal dose distribution. (*A*) Photon versus proton photon craniospinal irradiation dose distribution. Note dose to anterior organs of the thorax and abdomen. (*B*) Proton craniospinal irradiation completely spares anterior structures.

SUMMARY

Many patients with advanced cancer benefit from PRT, and consultation with a radiation oncologist should be considered for any patient with pain, bleeding, local complications, or other tumor-related symptoms. Although multiple techniques and dose-fractionation schemes may be appropriate for a given clinical presentation, some common situations, such as BM, cord compression, bone metastases, and poorly controlled primary tumors, have published series or RCTs to support varied PRT regimens. Multidisciplinary discussion remains of utmost importance in deciding on an integrated treatment regimen. PRT may be an effective alternative to surgical management in cases where resection would be highly morbid, technically challenging, or not feasible.

CLINICS CARE POINTS

- Validated prognostic tools should be used for multidisciplinary decision-making for palliative radiotherapy (PRT).
- Advanced cancers of primary sites have many options for palliation ranging from single fraction to conventionally fractionated treatment over several weeks.

- Surgery should be considered for solitary or symptomatic brain metastasis. Whole-brain radiotherapy (WBRT) has been the standard management option for decades, but modern paradigms are expanding indications for use of stereotactic radiosurgery and hippocampal avoidance WBRT.

- Uncomplicated bone metastases are best treated with single-fraction PRT with response rates ranging from 60% to 80%. Patients requiring retreatment can have 50% response rates.

- Multiple models exist to guide management of metastatic epidural spinal cord compression. Patients managed with upfront surgery should receive postoperative radiation, whereas patients managed without surgery can be treated with 1, 5, or 10 fractions of PRT.

- Certain clinical scenarios may benefit from more aggressive palliative radiation for local control, which may be considered to be disease-modifying and palliative. Advanced technologies may be appropriate.

REFERENCES

1. Murphy JD, Nelson LM, Chang DT, et al. Patterns of care in palliative radiotherapy: a population-based study. J Oncol Pract 2013;9(5):e220–7.
2. McDonald R, Ding K, Brundage M, et al. Effect of radiotherapy on painful bone metastases: a secondary analysis of the NCIC clinical trials group symptom control trial SC.23. JAMA Oncol 2017;3(7):953–9.
3. Katsoulakis E, Kumar K, Laufer I, et al. Stereotactic body radiotherapy in the treatment of spinal metastases. Semin Radiat Oncol 2017;27(3):209–17.
4. Laufer I, Rubin DG, Lis E, et al. The NOMS framework: approach to the treatment of spinal metastatic tumors. Oncologist 2013;18(6):744–51.
5. Tsao MN, Rades D, Wirth A, et al. Radiotherapeutic and surgical management for newly diagnosed brain metastasis(es): an American Society for Radiation Oncology evidence-based guideline. Pract Radiat Oncol 2012;2(3):210–25.
6. Rades D, Kasmann L, Schild SE, et al. A survival score for patients receiving palliative irradiation for locally advanced lung cancer. Clin Lung Cancer 2016;17(6): 558–62.
7. Sperduto PW, Kased N, Roberge D, et al. Summary report on the graded prognostic assessment: an accurate and facile diagnosis-specific tool to estimate survival for patients with brain metastases. J Clin Oncol 2012;30(4):419–25.
8. Cheon S, Agarwal A, Popovic M, et al. The accuracy of clinicians' predictions of survival in advanced cancer: a review. Ann Palliat Med 2016;5(1):22–9.
9. Mojica-Marquez AE, Rodriguez-Lopez JL, Patel AK, et al. External validation of life expectancy prognostic models in patients evaluated for palliative radiotherapy at the end-of-life. Cancer Med 2020;9(16):5781–7.
10. Alcorn SR, Fiksel J, Wright JL, et al. Developing an improved statistical approach for survival estimation in bone metastases management: the Bone Metastases Ensemble Trees for Survival (BMETS) model. Int J Radiat Oncol Biol Phys 2020;108(3):554–63.
11. Zylla D, Steele G, Gupta P. A systematic review of the impact of pain on overall survival in patients with cancer. Support Care Cancer 2017;25(5):1687–98.
12. Seong J, Park HC, Kim J, et al. Radiation-induced alteration of pain-related signals in an animal model with bone invasion from cancer. Ann N Y Acad Sci 2004; 1030:179–86.
13. Lutz S, Balboni T, Jones J, et al. Palliative radiation therapy for bone metastases: update of an ASTRO evidence-based guideline. Pract Radiat Oncol 2017; 7(1):4–12.

14. Vuong S, Pulenzas N, DeAngelis C, et al. Inadequate pain management in cancer patients attending an outpatient palliative radiotherapy clinic. Support Care Cancer 2016;24(2):887–92.

15. Johnstone C, Rich SE. Bleeding in cancer patients and its treatment: a review. Ann Palliat Med 2018;7(2):265–73.

16. Cihoric N, Crowe S, Eychmuller S, et al. Clinically significant bleeding in incurable cancer patients: effectiveness of hemostatic radiotherapy. Radiat Oncol 2012; 7:132.

17. Verheij M, Dewit LG, Boomgaard MN, et al. Ionizing radiation enhances platelet adhesion to the extracellular matrix of human endothelial cells by an increase in the release of von Willebrand factor. Radiat Res 1994;137(2):202–7.

18. Grewal AS, Freedman GM, Jones JA, et al. Hypofractionated radiation therapy for durable palliative treatment of bleeding, fungating breast cancers. Pract Radiat Oncol 2019;9(2):73–6.

19. Kondoh C, Shitara K, Nomura M, et al. Efficacy of palliative radiotherapy for gastric bleeding in patients with unresectable advanced gastric cancer: a retrospective cohort study. BMC Palliat Care 2015;14:37.

20. Eleje GU, Eke AC, Igberase GO, et al. Palliative interventions for controlling vaginal bleeding in advanced cervical cancer. Cochrane Database Syst Rev 2015;(5):CD011000.

21. Cameron MG, Kersten C, Vistad I, et al. Palliative pelvic radiotherapy of symptomatic incurable rectal cancer: a systematic review. Acta Oncol 2014;53(2): 164–73.

22. Cameron MG, Kersten C, Guren MG, et al. Palliative pelvic radiotherapy of symptomatic incurable prostate cancer: a systematic review. Radiother Oncol 2014; 110(1):55–60.

23. Vuong W, Lin J, Wei RL. Palliative radiotherapy for skin malignancies. Ann Palliat Med 2017;6(2):165–72.

24. Hanna TP, Shafiq J, Delaney GP, et al. The population benefit of evidence-based radiotherapy: 5-year local control and overall survival benefits. Radiother Oncol 2018;126(2):191–7.

25. Grewal AS, Jones J, Lin A. Palliative radiation therapy for head and neck cancers. Int J Radiat Oncol Biol Phys 2019;105(2):254–66.

26. Rodrigues G, Videtic GM, Sur R, et al. Palliative thoracic radiotherapy in lung cancer: an American Society for Radiation Oncology evidence-based clinical practice guideline. Pract Radiat Oncol 2011;1(2):60–71.

27. Stevens R, Macbeth F, Toy E, et al. Palliative radiotherapy regimens for patients with thoracic symptoms from non-small cell lung cancer. Cochrane Database Syst Rev 2015;1:CD002143.

28. Moeller B, Balagamwala EH, Chen A, et al. Palliative thoracic radiation therapy for non-small cell lung cancer: 2018 update of an American Society for Radiation Oncology (ASTRO) evidence-based guideline. Pract Radiat Oncol 2018;8(4): 245–50.

29. Simone CB 2nd, Bogart JA, Cabrera AR, et al. Radiation therapy for small cell lung cancer: an ASTRO clinical practice guideline. Pract Radiat Oncol 2020; 10(3):158–73.

30. Vempati P, Knoll MA, Dharmarajan K, et al. Palliation of ulcerative breast lesions with radiation. Anticancer Res 2016;36(9):4701–5.

31. Martin EJ, Bruggeman AR, Nalawade VV, et al. Palliative radiotherapy versus esophageal stent placement in the management of patients with metastatic esophageal cancer. J Natl Compr Canc Netw 2020;18(5):569–74.

32. Javed A, Pal S, Dash NR, et al. Palliative stenting with or without radiotherapy for inoperable esophageal carcinoma: a randomized trial. J Gastrointest Cancer 2012;43(1):63–9.

33. Penniment MG, De Ieso PB, Harvey JA, et al. Palliative chemoradiotherapy versus radiotherapy alone for dysphagia in advanced oesophageal cancer: a multicentre randomised controlled trial (TROG 03.01). Lancet Gastroenterol Hepatol 2018;3(2):114–24.

34. Deressa BT, Tigeneh W, Bogale N, et al. Short-Course 2-dimensional radiation therapy in the palliative treatment of esophageal cancer in a developing country: a phase II study (Sharon Project). Int J Radiat Oncol Biol Phys 2020;106(1):67–72.

35. Fuccio L, Mandolesi D, Farioli A, et al. Brachytherapy for the palliation of dysphagia owing to esophageal cancer: a systematic review and meta-analysis of prospective studies. Radiother Oncol 2017;122(3):332–9.

36. Tey J, Choo BA, Leong CN, et al. Clinical outcome of palliative radiotherapy for locally advanced symptomatic gastric cancer in the modern era. Medicine (Baltimore) 2014;93(22):e118.

37. Tey J, Soon YY, Koh WY, et al. Palliative radiotherapy for gastric cancer: a systematic review and meta-analysis. Oncotarget 2017;8(15):25797–805.

38. Bae SH, Park W, Choi DH, et al. Palliative radiotherapy in patients with a symptomatic pelvic mass of metastatic colorectal cancer. Radiat Oncol 2011;6:52.

39. Duchesne GM, Bolger JJ, Griffiths GO, et al. A randomized trial of hypofractionated schedules of palliative radiotherapy in the management of bladder carcinoma: results of medical research council trial BA09. Int J Radiat Oncol Biol Phys 2000;47(2):379–88.

40. Ali A, Song YP, Mehta S, et al. Palliative radiation therapy in bladder cancer-importance of patient selection: a retrospective multicenter study. Int J Radiat Oncol Biol Phys 2019;105(2):389–93.

41. Gogna NK, Baxi S, Hickey B, et al. Split-course, high-dose palliative pelvic radiotherapy for locally progressive hormone-refractory prostate cancer. Int J Radiat Oncol Biol Phys 2012;83(2):e205–11.

42. Elledge CR, Beriwal S, Chargari C, et al. Radiation therapy for gynecologic malignancies during the COVID-19 pandemic: International expert consensus recommendations. Gynecol Oncol 2020;158(2):244–53.

43. Spanos WJ Jr, Perez CA, Marcus S, et al. Effect of rest interval on tumor and normal tissue response: a report of phase III study of accelerated split course palliative radiation for advanced pelvic malignancies (RTOG-8502). Int J Radiat Oncol Biol Phys 1993;25(3):399–403.

44. Yan J, Milosevic M, Fyles A, et al. A hypofractionated radiotherapy regimen (0-7-21) for advanced gynaecological cancer patients. Clin Oncol (R Coll Radiol) 2011;23(7):476–81.

45. Mukerji B, Baptiste C, Chen L, et al. Racial disparities in young women with endometrial cancer. Gynecol Oncol 2018;148(3):527–34.

46. Yoo W, Kim S, Huh WK, et al. Recent trends in racial and regional disparities in cervical cancer incidence and mortality in United States. PLoS One 2017;12(2):e0172548.

47. Tom MC, Joshi N, Vicini F, et al. The American Brachytherapy Society consensus statement on intraoperative radiation therapy. Brachytherapy 2019;18(3):242–57.

48. Chang DT, Amdur RJ, Morris CG, et al. Adjuvant radiotherapy for cutaneous melanoma: comparing hypofractionation to conventional fractionation. Int J Radiat Oncol Biol Phys 2006;66(4):1051–5.

49. Casali PG, Abecassis N, Aro HT, et al. Soft tissue and visceral sarcomas: ESMO-EURACAN clinical practice guidelines for diagnosis, treatment and follow-up. Ann Oncol 2018;29(Suppl 4):iv51–67.

50. Tween H, Peake D, Spooner D, et al. Radiotherapy for the palliation of advanced sarcomas-the effectiveness of radiotherapy in providing symptomatic improvement for advanced sarcomas in a single centre cohort. Healthcare (Basel) 2019;7(4):120.

51. Kalbasi A, Kamrava M, Chu FI, et al. A phase II trial of 5-day neoadjuvant radiotherapy for patients with high-risk primary soft tissue sarcoma. Clin Cancer Res 2020;26(8):1829–36.

52. Kim E, Jeans E, Shinohara ET, et al. Stereotactic body radiotherapy (SBRT) for metastatic and recurrent soft tissue and bone sarcomas. Int J Radiat Oncol Biol Phys 2017;99(2):E754.

53. Suh JH, Kotecha R, Chao ST, et al. Current approaches to the management of brain metastases. Nat Rev Clin Oncol 2020;17(5):279–99.

54. Agency for Healthcare Research and Quality. Radiation therapy for brain metastases: a systematic review 2020. Available at: https://effectivehealthcare.ahrq.gov/products/radiation-brain-metastases/protocol. Accessed September 21, 2020.

55. Sperduto PW, Mesko S, Li J, et al. Survival in patients with brain metastases: summary report on the updated diagnosis-specific graded prognostic assessment and definition of the eligibility quotient. J Clin Oncol 2020;38(32):3773–84.

56. Mahajan A, Ahmed S, McAleer MF, et al. Post-operative stereotactic radiosurgery versus observation for completely resected brain metastases: a single-centre, randomised, controlled, phase 3 trial. Lancet Oncol 2017;18(8):1040–8.

57. Andrews DW, Scott CB, Sperduto PW, et al. Whole brain radiation therapy with or without stereotactic radiosurgery boost for patients with one to three brain metastases: phase III results of the RTOG 9508 randomised trial. Lancet 2004; 363(9422):1665–72.

58. Kocher M, Soffietti R, Abacioglu U, et al. Adjuvant whole-brain radiotherapy versus observation after radiosurgery or surgical resection of one to three cerebral metastases: results of the EORTC 22952-26001 study. J Clin Oncol 2011; 29(2):134–41.

59. Bhatnagar AK, Flickinger JC, Kondziolka D, et al. Stereotactic radiosurgery for four or more intracranial metastases. Int J Radiat Oncol Biol Phys 2006;64(3): 898–903.

60. Routman DM, Bian SX, Diao K, et al. The growing importance of lesion volume as a prognostic factor in patients with multiple brain metastases treated with stereotactic radiosurgery. Cancer Med 2018;7(3):757–64.

61. Brown PD, Gondi V, Pugh S, et al. Hippocampal avoidance during whole-brain radiotherapy plus memantine for patients with brain metastases: phase III trial NRG Oncology CC001. J Clin Oncol 2020;38(10):1019–29.

62. Mulvenna P, Nankivell M, Barton R, et al. Dexamethasone and supportive care with or without whole brain radiotherapy in treating patients with non-small cell lung cancer with brain metastases unsuitable for resection or stereotactic radiotherapy (QUARTZ): results from a phase 3, non-inferiority, randomised trial. Lancet 2016;388(10055):2004–14.

63. Chow E, van der Linden YM, Roos D, et al. Single versus multiple fractions of repeat radiation for painful bone metastases: a randomised, controlled, non-inferiority trial. Lancet Oncol 2014;15(2):164–71.

64. Lawton AJ, Lee KA, Cheville AL, et al. Assessment and management of patients with metastatic spinal cord compression: a multidisciplinary review. J Clin Oncol 2019;37(1):61–71.

65. Rades D, Segedin B, Conde-Moreno AJ, et al. Radiotherapy with 4 Gy x 5 versus 3 Gy x 10 for metastatic epidural spinal cord compression: final results of the SCORE-2 trial (ARO 2009/01). J Clin Oncol 2016;34(6):597–602.

66. Hoskin PJ, Hopkins K, Misra V, et al. Effect of single-fraction vs multifraction radiotherapy on ambulatory status among patients with spinal canal compression from metastatic cancer: the SCORAD randomized clinical trial. JAMA 2019;322(21): 2084–94.

67. Palma DA, Olson R, Harrow S, et al. Stereotactic ablative radiotherapy for the comprehensive treatment of oligometastatic cancers: long-term results of the SABR-COMET phase II randomized trial. J Clin Oncol 2020;38(25):2830–8.

68. Parker CC, James ND, Brawley CD, et al. Radiotherapy to the primary tumour for newly diagnosed, metastatic prostate cancer (STAMPEDE): a randomised controlled phase 3 trial. Lancet 2018;392(10162):2353–66.

69. Li D, Zhu X, Wang H, et al. Should aggressive thoracic therapy be performed in patients with synchronous oligometastatic non-small cell lung cancer? A meta-analysis. J Thorac Dis 2017;9(2):310–7.

70. Slotman BJ, van Tinteren H, Praag JO, et al. Use of thoracic radiotherapy for extensive stage small-cell lung cancer: a phase 3 randomised controlled trial. Lancet 2015;385(9962):36–42.

71. You R, Liu YP, Huang PY, et al. Efficacy and safety of locoregional radiotherapy with chemotherapy vs chemotherapy alone in de novo metastatic nasopharyngeal carcinoma: a multicenter phase 3 randomized clinical trial. JAMA Oncol 2020;6(9):1345–52.

72. Ma J, Lok BH, Zong J, et al. Proton radiotherapy for recurrent or metastatic head and neck cancers with palliative quad shot. Int J Part Ther 2018;4(4):10–9.

73. Liam CK. Central nervous system activity of first-line osimertinib in epidermal growth factor receptor-mutant advanced non-small cell lung cancer. Ann Transl Med 2019;7(3):61.

74. Phillips R, Shi WY, Deek M, et al. Outcomes of observation vs stereotactic ablative radiation for oligometastatic prostate cancer: the ORIOLE phase 2 randomized clinical trial. JAMA Oncol 2020;6(5):650–9.

75. Gomez DR, Tang C, Zhang J, et al. Local consolidative therapy vs. maintenance therapy or observation for patients with oligometastatic non-small-cell lung cancer: long-term results of a multi-institutional, phase II, randomized study. J Clin Oncol 2019;37(18):1558–65.

76. Iyengar P, Wardak Z, Gerber DE, et al. Consolidative radiotherapy for limited metastatic non-small-cell lung cancer: a phase 2 randomized clinical trial. JAMA Oncol 2018;4(1):e173501.

77. Palma DA, Olson R, Harrow S, et al. Stereotactic ablative radiotherapy versus standard of care palliative treatment in patients with oligometastatic cancers (SABR-COMET): a randomised, phase 2, open-label trial. Lancet 2019; 393(10185):2051–8.

78. Palma DA, Olson R, Harrow S, et al. Stereotactic ablative radiotherapy for the comprehensive treatment of 4-10 oligometastatic tumors (SABR-COMET-10): study protocol for a randomized phase III trial. BMC Cancer 2019;19(1):816.

Ethical Considerations in Caring for Patients with Advanced Malignancy

Alyssa K. Ovaitt, MD[a], Susan McCammon, MFA, MD[a,b,*]

KEYWORDS

- Palliative care • Ethics • Prognostication • Directive counsel • Affective forecasting
- Decisional regret • Therapeutic misconception • Nonabandonment

KEY POINTS

- Prognostication can shift into directive counsel, or trying to influence our patient to choose what we think is "right."
- Affective forecasting, or the way one will feel in the future after a decision made in the present, can help us to understand and mitigate the risks of decisional regret.
- Therapeutic misconception, or a patient misunderstanding that occurs when they do not distinguish between clinical research and their therapeutic treatment plan, must be explained, without taking away hope.
- The values of patient ownership and nonabandonment can be balanced with the interprofessional roles of palliative and curative intent.

INTRODUCTION

Advanced cancer, as defined by the National Cancer Institute, is "cancer that is unlikely to be cured or controlled with treatment… may have spread from where it first started to nearby tissue, lymph nodes, or distant parts of the body."[1] Some patients who carry this diagnosis may be just discovering the news for the first time, with their disease considered advanced on presentation, or they may have recurrent disease.

The authors have nothing to disclose.
[a] Department of Otolaryngology–Head and Neck Surgery, The University of Alabama at Birmingham, Faculty Office Tower 1155, 1720 2nd Avenue South, Birmingham, AL 35294-3412, USA; [b] Department of Internal Medicine, Division of Gerontology, Geriatrics, and Palliative Care, Community-Based Palliative Care, UAB Center for Palliative and Supportive Care, The University of Alabama at Birmingham, Faculty Office Tower 1155, 1720 2nd Avenue South, Birmingham, AL 35294-3412, USA
* Corresponding author. Department of Internal Medicine, Division of Gerontology, Geriatrics and Palliative Care, Community-Based Palliative Care, UAB Center for Palliative and Supportive Care, The University of Alabama at Birmingham, Faculty Office Tower 1155, 1720 2nd Avenue South, Birmingham, AL 35294-3412.
E-mail address: smccammon@uabmc.edu

Although such patients may have much in common, they also face different challenges or fears and have different needs from their providers. For instance, a patient who receives the news that their cancer is advanced upon their first presentation may question their own mortality or experience guilt about ignoring symptoms or persisting in high-risk behaviors. They may even feel anger at prior providers for missed diagnoses. Those dealing with recurrence may experience decisional regret or may belabor past decisions that have led to their current status, feel frustration and anger at a failed treatment (particularly if it was morbid), and trepidation about their remaining options that may include heroic surgery or palliative chemotherapy or immunotherapy.

As we encounter patients with advanced malignancy, it is critical that we are aware of the bioethical frameworks that guide our conversations and work. Ethics, after all, is the study or practice of determining right and wrong decisions or actions. Here, we present a case illustrating the many challenges of a patient with advanced cancer, followed by guided discussion about ethics that influence his treatment. In applying ethics to practice for patients with advanced malignancy, we can provide appropriate counsel without relying on prognostication alone, can assist our patients in avoiding decisional regret, can eliminate therapeutic misconception in those eligible for clinical trials, and can participate fully in patient care in solitary or as a part of a team that "shares" care.

DISCUSSION
Act 1

Mr Smith is a 49-year-old man with a history of stage III human papilloma virus–related squamous cell carcinoma of the right tonsil. He was referred for robotic surgical resection and neck dissection, which he underwent without complication. Unfortunately, his final pathology showed multiple positive lymph nodes with aggressive features as well as close margins. Thus, he was referred for adjuvant chemoradiation, which he tolerated with great difficulty, owing to the development of grade 4 mucositis and dysphagia requiring gastrostomy tube placement. He has struggled to regain his strength and control his pain so that he can return to work and his normal life with his partner and 2 small children. Recently, he feels he is getting worse, with increased pain and worsened swallowing. A PET scan is concerning for locoregional recurrence. He now has aggressive spread of recurrent disease at the primary site with necrotic lymphadenopathy in the contralateral neck, both biopsy-confirmed squamous cell carcinoma. Treatment options at this point are surgical salvage, which would include pharyngectomy, near total glossectomy, possible laryngectomy, and bilateral neck dissection with free flap reconstruction possibly followed by re-irradiation with protons; palliative chemotherapy; immunotherapy; supportive care without disease modifying treatment; and/or participation in a clinical trial.

His past medical history is significant for hypertension, clinical depression, and anxiety, but he has otherwise been healthy and athletic. He is an executive at a local company and has 2 small children with his partner, with close extended families in the area. As he sits in his surgeon's office, he absorbs this news and grapples with the decisions that will need to be made. These are the things that are in his mind.

Prognostication versus directive counsel

How we frame medical decisions depends greatly on how we understand the patient's disease trajectory and prognosis. Biomedical ethics exists within a larger framework of ethical systems dominated by consequentialism (utilitarian decisions should be made to optimize results) and deontology (Kantian, or duty-based ethics, where decisions are guided by absolute rules). In the medical world, consequentialism parallels outcomes-based research and practice: you should do what results in the best out-comes, focusing on rates of survival and quality of life. In contrast, deontological or duty-based ethics aim to identify a gold standard of care that is offered equitably to everyone or to respect a patient's wishes regardless of an anticipated outcome. Although a physician may use both frameworks or seem to favor one in an effort to do what they feel is best for their patient, the way we describe an outcome surely affects how our patients make choices.

Prognostication can be quite challenging owing to variability among advanced tumors and patients, as well as the ever changing medical treatment options and recommendations.[2] Beyond the survival curves and recommendations that exist, one must also use functional status, patient signs and symptoms, and quality of life, as well as one's own clinical experience to guide estimates.[2,3] Many studies have attempted to assess clinician's abilities to accurately predict prognosis, and find that values are frequently incorrect and often overestimated.[4–6] Mr Smith faces the challenge of choosing between multiple avenues of treatment, all of which carry their own negative ramifications. Not only has he already had a poorer outcome than predicted, but he now needs additional prognostication for each treatment choice, so that he can make an informed decision. It is understandable that the way these options are por-trayed will ultimately influence his decision.

Beyond the outcome that we suspect or how we arrive there, the way we disclose such information also sways how patients make choices. We may be tempted to adjust this description to encourage our patient to choose what we think is "right," also known as directive counseling.[7] Many have argued that this should not occur, given physician values may outweigh a patient's, while others propose that both physician and patient values should be weighed into such a choice.[8–10] Putman and colleagues[8] explored this question, finding that most primary physicians report they avoid directive counsel when medical decisions are "morally controversial."[9] Ulti-mately, guidelines about how to have these conversations is lacking, and it is up to the physician and patient to determine how best to guide or make such decisions. Sharing physician experience and knowledge while not imposing personal bias is a balance that we should likely always continue to explore and improve.

Act 2

When he was initially diagnosed with tonsil cancer, he was told this was a "good" can-cer to have. His understanding was that the p16 marker meant that he would respond well to treatment, so well in fact that research was showing ways to decrease the in-tensity of treatment to cure the cancer with less severe side effects. His doctor advised him to travel to a major cancer center to have robotic surgery in the hopes he might not have to have radiation at all, much less chemotherapy. He was under-standably disappointed when the surgeon who did his robotic surgery told him that his tissue had bad features that predicted a poorer prognosis, and that he would need to have radiation and chemotherapy in addition to the painful surgery he had already had. His surgeon wanted him to be treated at the big center, but this was far from home and he successfully negotiated permission to get chemoradiation in his hometown.

His postoperative treatment was much worse than anticipated, but he was moti-vated to do everything he could to ensure long-term survival so that he could continue to raise his children. When thinking about his future, he felt sure that any price (eg, discomfort or change in eating or speaking) would be worth long-term survival. After the severe side effects of adjuvant chemoradiation and now facing a radical resection and reconstruction, he has begun to doubt himself quietly. He still wants to be aggressive in his treatment course, but he is afraid of disfigurement and unintelligible speech. He begins to wonder if he made a mistake in his original treatment decisions. His clinical depression, previously controlled with counseling and medication, re-emerges.

Affective forecasting and decisional regret

The weight of affective forecasting, or a patient's prediction of how one will feel in the future about a decision one is making in the present, should not be underesti-mated.[11,12] Given the course and nature of advanced cancer management, numerous simple and complex decisions will be required throughout the disease course. Often, particularly with decisions that will affect their quality of life, patients poorly predict how they will adapt to the scenario of their choosing.[13] Some studies have identified cognitive biases that contribute to poor affective forecasting, such as focalism, im-mune neglect, impact bias, and failure to predict adaptation.[11,13,14] Ellis and col-leagues[11] lists 4 main features of palliative care that contribute to poor affective predictions: intense emotions, involvement of multiple people in decision-making, the decision or cancer's effect on the patient's life beyond their physical health (eg, relationships), and inadequate prognostic information. Still other investigators have focused on factors like personality traits that may contribute to patients making more accurate predictions and realistic paradigms.[12,15] As clinicians, we can assist by recognizing when biases may be occurring, being clear about our prognostic pre-dictions, and limiting the additional stigmas, emotional distress, and clinician bias that may add to the already challenging decision.[13]

Once the decision has been made, patients may also face decisional regret if they later feel that they made the wrong choice, particularly if the choice was a difficult one or if the choice will affect their function or quality of life.[16] As in this case example, pa-tients with recurrent cancer may experience regret about their decision in retrospect. In choosing a certain treatment course, regardless of the odds or discussions at that time, the patient changes their disease trajectory when they make a choice. Several studies, including those on prostate cancer and oropharyngeal cancer, suggest that quality of life outcomes and persistent symptoms after treatment promote decisional regret.[16,17] Fully explaining the side effects or consequences of treatment choices on quality of life, as well as treating post-treatment symptoms, are helpful strategies to decrease decisional regret.[16] Decisional regret may also make a patient feel impaired when trying to make their next decision, belaboring the analysis of options and affec-tive forecasting. In this case, Mr Smith experiences doubt about future treatment as well as regret about his previous choice that led to his significant pain and difficulty swallowing. Affective forecasting and imagining further decline in his quality of life, while weighing his familial obligations and ultimate goals, are all important discussion points in his decision.

In such instances, it may behoove the clinician to discuss the nature of these com-plex decisions with their patient. With any decision, unsupported or unfettered auton-omy and the need to make any significant decision alone will inevitably lead to doubt, if not frank regret. Understanding the patient's experience and its effect on their current risk tolerance can help to guide patient choice. For example, the patient with recurrent cancer despite primary surgical management in the past may be less threatened by systemic therapy than another aggressive salvage operation. This circumstance is in contrast with Mr Smith's case, who had substantial morbidity from his chemo-therapy and radiation, and is hesitant to consider any further treatments that may lead to additional functional decline. Here, recognizing the patient's internal story arc may help.[18] Mr Smith, for example, was previously hoping for restitution to his prior normal state, and later when facing his recurrence, he is hoping to conceptualize his cancer treatment as a quest narrative to a new normal, which does not necessarily have to be worse than his previous state. There are many methods to assist complex decision-making and to avoid complications of it, with clear communication, understanding of the patient's narrative, and addressing decisional regret (if it occurs) at the forefront.

Act 3

Mr Smith tells his surgeon he wants to move directly to the most aggressive treatment possible; he states that he is willing to undergo experimental therapy and would like to be enrolled in a clinical trial. The only clinical trial he is eligible for is a phase I trial toxicity and safety trial and he becomes fixated on getting into the trial or getting the drug on a compassionate use exception. His surgeon advises him that this may not provide the best possible treatment for his recurrent cancer and he is concerned with the patient's emotional lability and worsening depression.

Therapeutic misconception

Therapeutic misconception occurs when a patient does not distinguish between clinical research and their therapeutic treatment plan, and thus fails to understand the differing goals of or the likelihood of benefit from their involvement in the research study.[19–22] Many factors contribute to therapeutic misconception, including inherent trust in the physician's aims, exaggeration of benefits portrayed by the media or others, a patient (or family's) desire to keep fighting, and/or a poor understanding about research among the lay public as a whole, among others.[22] Advanced cancer may also create a paradox between a patient's desperate interest in additional treatment options and a community's desperate need for clinical trials, with patients who carry a diagnosis of advanced malignancy often only eligible for phase I trials. Despite changes in early phase trials in recent years, patients may still fail to recognize that their study is assessing toxicity or dose escalation and is not expected to provide any disease-altering or personal benefit.[23,24] If a patient fails to recognize that their contribution may be more beneficial to future generations with advanced disease, rather than to themselves, they have fallen prey to therapeutic misconception; unfortunately, this phenomenon seems to be all too common.[25]

Regardless of the etiology, therapeutic misconception degrades the ethical and true definition of consent and may lead to great distrust among an already vulnerable population. To complicate this subject further, therapeutic misconception must also be balanced with a clinician's proclivity toward cultivating hope in patients with advanced cancer and promoting studies that have potential to help others as well. As in this case example, clinical trials can create ethical dilemmas in patients with advanced cancer, as many have already expunged curative treatment options and are desperate for "a miracle." In such patients, physicians may want to consider the patient's care circle in their decision-making and potential outcomes.

In patients with advanced cancer, for whom curative therapies have already been tried, the inclusion of a patient's caregivers within conversation may be critical to decision-making. Although it is the clinician/researcher's ethical responsibility to ensure a patient understands the true role of the clinical trial proposed (eg, who is truly undergoing treatment vs who is expected to benefit), they should also consider who will be responsible for managing patient toxicities and disappointment if side effects are encountered or no clinical benefit is seen, respectively. In patients who experience therapeutic optimism, meaning that they recognize that participating in a research trial may not actually treat their disease, but they greatly hope that it will,[22] it is especially important to consider opinions of involved parties before a patient enrolls. As with Mr Smith, trials can offer great hope to patients who are lacking additional options, and it is a physician's responsibility to explain therapeutic misconception and avoid it.

Act 4

The patient is referred to the palliative care clinic for a goals of care conversation and for help with coping with serious illness. The patient is unsure of what palliative care is, but is encouraged by the cheerful sign above the door that advertises "Supportive Care and Survivorship." The conversation, in his opinion, wanders to include his past and current life, his hopes and expectations, and how he is thinking about the recurrent cancer and the options he faces. He is able to share his doubts about the major surgery in a way that he did not feel he could share with his surgeon, but he is then dismayed when the palliative care doctor introduces the role of hospice in optimizing of the time that he has remaining. He leaves that clinic, unsure of who his primary doctor is now.

Professionalism in "sharing" care

Balancing patient ownership and nonabandonment can color the relationship between the surgical team and the palliative team.[26–32] A patient with an aggressive treating clinician who actively seeks out a palliative care consult may feel more able to express doubt about decisions to a third party. A hero surgeon/oncologist may feel torn between 2 sets of values: importance of preserving the original doctor patient relationship, with access and communication, while still providing safe space, liaison, with a different, neutral third party. There may be internal tension for a surgeon who transitions from a curative to a palliative intent with the same patient. Some people consider allowing radical autonomy that leads to goal-discordant care to be a kind of patient abandonment, especially when a patient winds up on life support in intensive care unit without plan for dependence on life-sustaining technology. Nonabandonment can be conflated with patient ownership. It becomes fraught, because surgeons can feel possessive of a patient and plan, but also can feel tremendous guilt over bad outcomes that they feel like they are the agent of. This can complicate recommendations, especially for end of life care.[31]

With increased training in both generalist and specialist palliative care among surgeons of all subspecialties, it is becoming more common for patients with advanced cancer to receive upstream palliative counseling.[33,34] The American Society of Clinical Oncology position statement on palliative care recommends that all patients who receive a diagnosis of advanced cancer receive a palliative care consultation at the point of diagnosis.[35]

In an ideal situation, Mr Smith's surgeon will have engaged him in discussions early on about the range of possible outcomes and subsequent decisions that may need to be made. Certainly, at the time that the recurrence is diagnosed, compassion and candor in addressing his doubts and apprehensions would be valuable. If he continues to grapple with his decision, consultation with a palliative care specialist can be introduced as a complementary service to aid him and his partner with articulating goals of care that can then lead to a goal-concordant decision that they can then discuss with their surgeon.

SUMMARY

Patients with advanced cancer, recurrent or at the time of diagnosis, face extraordinary challenges that raise ethical questions about care to the aware physician. How we prognosticate and then communicate with patients is the start of these challenges and should lead to shared decision making between care providers, family members, patients, and health care professionals. Anticipating how one will adapt to the outcomes of one's decisions is challenging but can help decision making and avoidance of decisional regret. We must also be aware of our own biases, in addition to our patients', when assisting with difficult or life-changing choices. Treatment may lead to hope in clinical trials, but therapeutic misconception should always be avoided, particularly with respect to patients at high risk for it and desperate for additional treatment options. As treatment decisions compound, patients may feel a sense of confusion or abandonment when visiting multiple providers, but they may also benefit from different spaces in which to share their concerns and hopes. Increased training in palliative care for surgeons can normalize some of the trepidation surrounding decision-making as treatment options narrow and possible outcomes become more limited. In remembering these entities within our main ethical framework, we can provide more effective and compassionate guidance to our patients already facing the daunting undertaking of living with advanced malignancy.

REFERENCES

1. Institute NC. NCI Dictionary of Cancer Terms. NIH. Available at: https://www.cancer.gov/publications/dictionaries/cancer-terms/. Accessed October 1, 2020.
2. Lamont EB, Christakis NA. Complexities in prognostication in advanced cancer: "to help them live their lives the way they want to. JAMA 2003;290(1):98–104.
3. Kelley AS, Morrison RS, Wenger NS, et al. Determinants of treatment intensity for patients with serious illness: a new conceptual framework. J Palliat Med 2010; 13(7):807–13.
4. Glare P, Virik K, Jones M, et al. A systematic review of physicians' survival predictions in terminally ill cancer patients. BMJ 2003;327(7408):195–8.
5. Amano K, Maeda I, Shimoyama S, et al. The accuracy of physicians' clinical predictions of survival in patients with advanced cancer. J Pain Symptom Manage 2015;50(2):139–146 e1.
6. Cheon S, Agarwal A, Popovic M, et al. The accuracy of clinicians' predictions of survival in advanced cancer: a review. Ann Palliat Med 2016;5(1):22–9.
7. McCammon SD. Concurrent palliative care in the surgical management of head and neck cancer. J Surg Oncol 2019;120(1):78–84.
8. Putman MS, Yoon JD, Rasinski KA, et al. Directive counsel and morally controversial medical decision-making: findings from two national surveys of primary care physicians. J Gen Intern Med 2014;29(2):335–40.
9. Yoon JD, Rasinski KA, Curlin FA. Moral controversy, directive counsel, and the doctor's role: findings from a national survey of obstetrician-gynecologists. Acad Med 2010;85(9):1475–81.
10. Zehnder NG. Capsule commentary on Putman et al., directive counsel and morally controversial medical decision-making: findings from two national surveys of primary care physicians. J Gen Intern Med 2014;29(2):361.
11. Ellis EM, Barnato AE, Chapman GB, et al. Toward a conceptual model of affective predictions in palliative care. J Pain Symptom Manage 2019;57(6):1151–65.
12. Hoerger M, Chapman B, Duberstein P. Realistic affective forecasting: the role of personality. Cogn Emot 2016;30(7):1304–16.
13. Halpern J, Arnold RM. Affective forecasting: an unrecognized challenge in making serious health decisions. J Gen Intern Med 2008;23(10):1708–12.

14. Wilson TD, Gilbert DT. Affective forecasting: knowing what to want. Curr Dir Psychol Sci 2005;14(3):131–4.

15. Funder DC. On the accuracy of personality judgment: a realistic approach. Psychol Rev 1995;102(4):652–70.

16. Goepfert RP, Fuller CD, Gunn GB, et al. Symptom burden as a driver of decisional regret in long-term oropharyngeal carcinoma survivors. Head Neck 2017;39(11): 2151–8.

17. Diefenbach MA, Mohamed NE. Regret of treatment decision and its association with disease-specific quality of life following prostate cancer treatment. Cancer Invest 2007;25(6):449–57.

18. Ratcliff C, Naik AD, Martin LA, et al. Examining cancer survivorship trajectories: exploring the intersection between qualitative illness narratives and quantitative screening instruments. Palliat Support Care 2018;16(6):712–8.

19. Jansen LA, Mahadevan D, Appelbaum PS, et al. Variations in unrealistic optimism between acceptors and decliners of early phase cancer trials. J Empir Res Hum Res Ethics 2017;12(4):280–8.

20. Appelbaum PS, Anatchkova M, Albert K, et al. Therapeutic misconception in research subjects: development and validation of a measure. Clin Trials Dec 2012;9(6):748–61.

21. Burke NJ. Rethinking the therapeutic misconception: social justice, patient advocacy, and cancer clinical trial recruitment in the US safety net. BMC Med Ethics 2014;15:68.

22. Grieselhuber NR, Kodner IJ, Brown D, et al. Confronting the therapeutic misconception. Surgery 2017;162(1):183–7.

23. Cassel JB, Del Fabbro E, Arkenau T, et al. Phase I cancer trials and palliative care: antagonism, irrelevance, or synergy? J Pain Symptom Manage 2016; 52(3):437–45.

24. Pentz RD, White M, Harvey RD, et al. Therapeutic misconception, misestimation, and optimism in participants enrolled in phase 1 trials. Cancer 2012;118(18): 4571–8.

25. Catt S, Langridge C, Fallowfield L, et al. Reasons given by patients for participating, or not, in Phase 1 cancer trials. Eur J Cancer 2011;47(10):1490–7.

26. Conn LG, Haas B, Cuthbertson BH, et al. Communication and culture in the surgical intensive care unit: boundary production and the improvement of patient care. Qual Health Res 2015.

27. Haas B, Gotlib Conn L, Rubenfeld GD, et al. "It's Parallel Universes": an analysis of communication between surgeons and intensivists. Crit Care Med 2015; 43(10):2147–54.

28. McLaren K, Lord J, Murray SB, et al. Ownership of patient care: a behavioural definition and stepwise approach to diagnosing problems in trainees. Perspect Med Educ 2013.

29. Paul Olson TJ, Brasel KJ, Redmann AJ, et al. Surgeon-reported conflict with intensivists about postoperative goals of care. JAMA Surg 2013;148(1):29–35.

30. Redmann AJ, Brasel KJ, Alexander CG, et al. Use of advance directives for high-risk operations: a national survey of surgeons. Ann Surg 2012;255(3):418–23.

31. Schwarze ML, Redmann AJ, Brasel KJ, et al. The role of surgeon error in withdrawal of postoperative life support. Ann Surg 2012;256(1):10–5.

32. Schwarze ML, Redmann AJ, Alexander GC, et al. Surgeons expect patients to buy-in to postoperative life support preoperatively: results of a national survey. Crit Care Med 2013;41(1):1–8.

33. Quill TE, Abernethy AP. Generalist plus specialist palliative care–creating a more sustainable model. The New Engl J Med 2013;368(13):1173–5.
34. Dunn GP. Surgical palliative care: recent trends and developments. Anesthesiol Clin 2012;30(1):13–28.
35. Ferrell BR, Temel JS, Temin S, et al. Integration of palliative care into standard oncology care: American Society of Clinical Oncology clinical practice guideline update. J Clin Oncol 2017;35(1):96–112.

Role of Palliative Medicine Training in Surgical Oncology

Alexandra C. Istl, MD, MPH, Fabian M. Johnston, MD, MHS*

KEYWORDS

- Palliative care • End of life • Palliative medicine training • Surgical education
- Surgical oncology • Fellowship

KEY POINTS

- Surgical oncologists should be well-versed in palliative and end-of-life care principles.
- Educational initiatives to improve palliative care skills among trainees and practitioners have been met with increasing interest and study in the last decade.
- Short-term didactic palliative care training interventions may not foster the critical reasoning necessary to provide optimal end-of-life care for patients with cancer.
- Developing active and immersive methods of palliative care education for trainees requires collaboration between surgical oncologists and palliative care physicians.
- There are many resources in print and online for trainees and practitioners seeking to improve their understanding of palliative care and end-of-life skills.

BACKGROUND

The benefit of integrating early palliative care (PC) into routine oncology practice has become well established over the last decade. With a growing interest in optimizing end-of-life (EOL) care, high-level evidence has emerged supporting the use of integrative PC and early palliative interventions. Numerous randomized trials in oncology have substantiated the value of early integrative PC, improving patient-centered outcomes such as depressive symptoms,[1,2] satisfaction with care,[3] decreased intravenous chemotherapy in final months of life,[4] and quality of life (QOL) on multiple validated QOL scales.[1-3] A 2010 randomized controlled trial of patients with advanced non–small cell lung carcinoma showed a 3.3-month improvement in median survival ($P = .02$) for patients enrolled in early PC versus standard care.[2] This finding is corroborated by a later trial evaluating patients with advanced solid or hematologic malignancies that demonstrated a 15% greater 1-year survival in patients for whom PC

Division of Surgical Oncology, Johns Hopkins Hospital, Blalock 684, 600 North Wolfe Street, Baltimore, MD 21287, USA
* Corresponding author.
E-mail address: fjohnst4@jhmi.edu
Twitter: @AllyIstl (A.C.I.); @FabianJohnston (F.M.J.)

Surg Oncol Clin N Am 30 (2021) 591–608
https://doi.org/10.1016/j.soc.2021.02.009
1055-3207/21/© 2021 Elsevier Inc. All rights reserved.

was implemented early.[5] Furthermore, patients with early PC had less aggressive measures taken at the end of life, increased use of hospice care, and better documentation of resuscitation preferences.[2]

Although surgeons contributed to the inception of PC and hospice, and it was a surgeon who coined the term "palliative care,"[6,7] the surgeon role in holistic EOL care for patients with advanced malignancies is often conspicuously absent. Surgeons are an invaluable asset in multidisciplinary PC and deploy an arsenal of surgical procedures to provide symptom management in patients with advanced cancer. Across specialties, surgeons now routinely perform procedures that allow basic activities such as nutritional intake, ambulation, and waste elimination to occur comfortably at the end of life. However, despite pervasive surgeon involvement in palliative procedures, surgeons lose opportunities to provide primary PC (i.e. fundamental symptom management and psychosocial care provided by a non-palliative medicine specialist) to patients with advanced malignancies. One of the biggest factors contributing to this deficit is the lack of formal education highlighting the value of multidisciplinary PC and the surgeon's role on that team.

The World Health Organization, describing PC as a physical, psychosocial, and spiritual approach to the end of life, cites a number of aims and objectives that can be used to guide PC educational initiatives for oncology practitioners.[8] These goals include providing pain and symptom relief, affirmation of life, and support systems for patients and families. The World Health Organization also advocates that PC is best delivered early and as a multidisciplinary team.[8] The executive summary from the 2000 National Consensus Conference on Medical Education for Care Near End of Life identified 9 domains relevant to PC education. These domains include pain and symptom management, psychosocial care, patient–physician communication about the end of life, and clinical experience in hospice or PC rotations.[9,10] Some of these have been adopted into the Accreditation Council for Graduate Medical Education postgraduate program requirements. However, no program includes all PC domains as a requisite part of training and surgical programs in particular incorporate very few.[9] With published objectives readily available, and in light of recommendations for and the known benefit of early PC, training programs should do more to incorporate formal PC education into their curricula.

This article reviews the evidence pertaining to PC training and education in surgical postgraduate education and practice. We identify gaps in the literature and present avenues for future study in PC education. Resources for surgical oncologists and trainees seeking additional formal training in PC are presented at the end of the article.

CURRENT EVIDENCE IN EDUCATION

The importance of EOL education is loosely reflected in undergraduate medical training. Although highly variable in its extent and mode of delivery,[11,12] EOL care is now incorporated into all undergraduate curricula in North America.[11] It is also reflected in the International Association of Medical Colleges' Liaison Committee on Medical Education composite standards, which require that all students starting medical school after June 1, 2000, undergo training in pain management and EOL care.[13] However, there are no specifications as to how this training should be implemented. The strength of a well-designed undergraduate curriculum would likely be measured by broad foundational principles, targeted to include EOL care for patients with cancer, chronic disease, and acute life-threatening illnesses. However, oncology patients have specific and nuanced PC needs that differ from patients with other chronic diseases; the necessity of oncology-specific PC training at the surgical residency, fellowship, and practice levels cannot be overstated.

Postgraduate Training

Residency

Evidence for PC training in residency programs has only recently started to include surgical trainees. In a 2019 systematic review of trials assessing postgraduate PC education interventions, only 2 of 6 trials included surgical residents,[14,15] and only 1 of those trials evaluated PC training for surgery residents exclusively.[15] For many residents, the absence of a PC curriculum represents an unmet training objective: multiple surveys of surgical residents have demonstrated a desire for further PC training. In a 2007 study from Brown University assessing the impact of a PC curriculum specifically for general surgery residents, almost all participants agreed that all surgical training programs should include a course on PC and EOL issues. Study results demonstrated that residents' confidence in breaking bad news and speaking to patients about EOL issues improved after completing a 3-day curriculum.[16] In a 2019 survey of residents from the Oregon Health and Sciences University, 100% of respondents wanted additional education in delivering bad news, discussing comfort-focused care, and leading goals-of-care conferences.[17] Of those surveyed, 85% wanted a formal PC curriculum to be included in their residency education.[17] Faculty corroborated these views, with 90% to 94% of faculty believing residents would benefit from such training. However, despite eagerness for additional education, more than half of the residents reported that they already felt comfortable leading conferences delivering bad news and discussing comfort-focused care and goals of care. This finding demonstrates some inconsistency between training experience and trainee confidence.

Similar confidence was documented in a 2010 trial of PC education.[15] The intervention group consisted of postgraduate year (PGY) 2 residents undergoing a 6-hour PC curriculum intervention focusing on ethical issues, patient and family support, critical appraisal of the literature, breaking bad news, and conducting family meetings.[15] This was the first year the curriculum had been implemented; no higher level residents had been exposed. PGY 2 residents showed a 9% improvement between their preintervention and postintervention multiple-choice question test, but neither their postintervention test scores nor their objective structured clinical examination results were better than the PGY 5 resident control group. Furthermore, they felt significantly less comfortable than the PGY 5 group in managing pain, breaking bad news, and addressing ethical issues with patients and families, even after the educational intervention.[15] All participants in the PGY 5 group felt comfortable breaking bad news and addressing ethical issues and 83% felt comfortable managing pain, nonpain symptoms, terminal care, and hospice transfer, despite none having formal education in PC. One-half of the PGY 5 cohort and 57% of the PGY 2 cohort believed that surgery residents receive adequate PC training through clinical experience. Similar to other studies included in the review, the main outcomes used to measure success of the intervention were resident recall and confidence with EOL care and conversations. Although confidence is important, this choice of outcomes warrants some discussion. The progression of surgical training provides an excellent analogy for this; being able to describe the steps of an operation and feeling confident in one's ability to cut and sew does not mean a surgical trainee can do a Whipple independently. Even for procedures that surgical trainees become comfortable performing independently (e.g. laparoscopic cholecystectomy), the attending surgeon frequently has suggestions that will improve the ease and safety of the operation.

Data from outside oncology suggest that provider comfort and experience do not necessarily translate into an accurate assessment of patient preferences. One study demonstrated that neither interns' nor attending physicians' understanding of their patients' preferences was congruent with their patients' actual wishes.[18] Physician perception of patient preference versus actual patient preference was evaluated for patient willingness to tolerate several adverse outcomes related to chronic illness: life-long tube feeding, chronic pain, chronic confusion, ventilator dependence, permanent coma, and transition to a nursing home. A weighted κ-statistic showed no agreement between physician perception and actual patient goals (beyond that which could explained by chance) for any adverse events except living in a nursing home, for which the κ-statistic showed fair agreement ($\kappa = 0.37$).[18] Within oncology, a recent study surveyed oncology inpatients about their understanding of advance care planning (ACP) and their preferences for engaging in those discussions.[19] Patients reported that rushed conversations, perceived ineffective interpersonal skills, and a lack of cultural competency deterred patients from wanting to engage in ACP discussions with their surgeon or oncologist. This finding may further support the conclusion that physician experience managing life-threatening diseases and physician confidence engaging in EOL and PC discussions, although important, do not ensure successful EOL or ACP conversations or palliation. Just as complex surgical procedures tend to have better outcomes in the hands of a high-volume surgeon, improved EOL outcomes are reasonably achieved in the hands of a PC-trained clinician, and we should be striving to integrate and ingrain formal PC training into our postgraduate curricula.

As we incorporate formal PC education into our postgraduate curricula, what outcomes will determine whether the educational initiatives we adopt are successful? The success of educational interventions is often judged either by testing students on curriculum material or assessing their confidence in applying course content (as discussed elsewhere in this article). By evaluating them in this way, we are usually trying to ascertain whether students have successfully learned the relevant principles and can apply them to a variety of clinical scenarios in a thoughtful, academic, and empathetic way. Confidence and information recall are important for resident performance; there is valuable literature emphasizing that involvement in a PC curriculum improves trainee confidence.[20] Similarly, a lack of formal training in PC and EOL discussions leads to poorer trainee confidence in their ability to communicate with patients about these issues.[20,21] However, there is also evidence that trainees' self-assessment of their communication skills does not correspond with patient or family assessments of the same interactions.[22] Internal medicine residents and fellows assessed their own communication skills on two quality of communication scales, including one focused on EOL communication. Patients and families evaluated them on the same scales and no positive associations were found. In fact, high trainee self-assessments were associated with low family assessments when engaging in treatment discussions ($P<.01$).[22] These studies provide further evidence that, as outcome measures, confidence and the ability to recall information do not necessarily reflect the critical reasoning skills we hope to cultivate in PC training programs.

Applying PC principles in an evidence-based fashion in surgical training and practice often requires physicians to challenge dogmas in other areas of their practice. They have to think critically and differently about the goals of PC and the available avenues for ensuring comfort both at the EOL and even earlier for patients with life limiting illness. As the PC education study in surgical trainees demonstrated, PGY 2 residents receiving PC education who showed good knowledge recall still had difficulty applying that knowledge clinically and remained uncomfortable doing so.[15] Trainees should be able to understand the unique nature of PC principles and critically evaluate how these learned principles apply to each patient they encounter. Ideally, PC education intervention studies would examine outcomes that reflect this cognitive and clinical development.

In 2012, a workgroup composed of a PC physician/psycho-oncologist, an educational psychologist, and an acute care surgeon/intensivist developed a PC curriculum based on the American College of Surgeons manual: *Surgical Palliative Care: A Resident's Guide*.[23] They created an objective educational assessment tool that was designed to measure participant attitude changes toward PC applications in surgery.[24] This survey tool was used again in a 2017 study to evaluate a new PC education program for general surgery residents, where participants took the survey both before and after the intervention, as well as 5 months later.[25] In the 2012 study, participant postintervention responses were significantly more consistent with PC best practice for several of the attitudes explored, including understanding and management of malignant small bowel obstruction and timing of PC initiation. However, attitudes less consistent with PC best practice were observed for items including delirium management and the impact of talking to a patient about dying.[24] In the 2017 study, there was an overall significant positive move toward expressing attitudes consistent with best practice PC.[25] However, although individual survey items showed improvement in attitudes consistent with PC principles, there were several items that showed underwhelming improvement after the educational intervention. Despite this finding, almost all residents agreed or strongly agreed that they felt comfortable having discussions pertaining to prognosis, EOL care, and PC options after the intervention.[25] This study further suggests that trainee or provider confidence and comfort does not always reflect a true understanding of clinical principles and best practice.

The objective assessment tool used in these studies was designed to evaluate the residents' capacity to critically evaluate their PC teaching and apply it to PC statements, yet the findings confirm the need for better interventions to provide consistent education. These findings may also be driven by pragmatic considerations that must be accounted for when developing educational interventions. These considerations include time constraints in residency education and the failure of traditional didactics to educate residents effectively in providing primary PC. There is a need for interdisciplinary time-condensed PC curricula that go beyond a simple series of lectures, but are succinct enough to fit into the busy surgical resident schedule. That being stated, similar to most things in medicine, experiential training is imperative to produce competent residents. A formal assessment by surgeons trained in PC domains or a formal PC rotation as a part of an inpatient and outpatient interdisciplinary team may be necessary to give surgical residents the formal instruction, supervised practice, and integrative understanding of resources and options they require to deliver PC properly.

Clinical fellowship

Fellows in surgical oncology are involved daily in both inpatient and outpatient discussions about disease course, prognosis, goals of care, and procedures for symptom management. They then coordinate those procedures, monitor patients after interventions, and manage the complications of those interventions, often with frequent follow-up in clinic and in hospital. Furthermore, in contrast with residency, surgical oncology fellows are exclusively managing patients with malignancy. EOL conversations and PC during residency are often directed at emergency surgery patients with significant comorbidities, patients with severe postoperative complications, critically ill patients in the intensive care unit, and trauma patients with devastating injuries. Patients with cancer and their families have unique needs and unique options available to them including systemic therapy and clinical trials, so the PC knowledge required of cancer care providers will also be unique. Even fellows who had robust PC training in residency may not be fully equipped upon entering fellowship to discuss such options and provide optimal palliation to patients with cancer. Given the institutional differences in care pathways, allied health services, and state and provincial variations in resources, it is reasonable to assume that additional interdisciplinary PC training would benefit even PC-literate surgical oncology fellows.

Recent surveys have assessed the frequency of PC skills teaching in surgical oncology, hepatopancreaticobiliary oncology, and gynecologic oncology clinical fellowships. These studies used similar instruments to explore how frequently faculty provided fellows with explicit education on a number of PC clinical skills: referral to PC teams, rotating opioid medications, treating neuropathic pain versus other pain sources, assessing and managing depression, discussing cessation of antineoplastic therapy and changing to a PC focus, telling a patient they are dying, helping families with reconciliation, and managing the personal stress arising from the provision of EOL care.[26–28]

The 2 survey studies of American gynecologic oncology fellows in 2013 and 2014 reported similar outcomes: survey respondents reported explicit teaching on neuropathic pain in approximately 31% and 27% of programs, respectively, and explicit teaching on rotating opioids in 17% and 20% of programs, respectively.[27,28] However, the reported frequencies for explicit teaching of other skills were low. Fewer than 20% of American gynecologic oncology fellows in both cohorts reported explicit teaching in managing patients' depression, handling personal stress in caring for terminally ill patients, and helping patients and families to reconcile.[27,28] Only hospice referral and cessation of antineoplastic therapy discussions were taught more frequently, with explicit teaching on hospice referral reported by 49% and 50% in the 2013 and 2014 studies, respectively, and stopping antineoplastic therapy in 52% and 57%, respectively.[27,28] In the 2013 survey, only 4 of 103 respondents had completed a PC rotation and, when asked about preparedness for practice, a PC rotation or other high-volume PC exposure were the only factors independently associated with self-reported readiness for clinical EOL care.[28] In the 2014 cohort, the number of discussions fellows led on changing goals of care, as well as attendings observing and providing feedback on those discussions, were associated with increased overall preparedness for EOL care in practice ($P<.0005$). However, 56% of respondents reported never receiving feedback on this skill.[27]

Teaching in pain management measures were not reported for hepatopancreaticobiliary/surgical oncology fellows. Only 32% reported explicit teaching for referring patients to hospice, 27% for stopping antineoplastic therapy, 20% for managing personal stress, 19% for telling a patient they are dying, and 14% for assisting families with reconciliation.[26] Despite infrequent formal education in these skills, 93% of US hepatopancreaticobiliary/surgical oncology fellows reported assessing pain in their most recent patient encounter, 85% had discussed goals of therapy, 50% had discussed psychosocial issues, and 48% had discussed dying with the patient.[26] Thirty-one percent of fellows reported that EOL care education was very good or excellent in their program, but more than one-half of fellows had never been observed or received feedback about their approach to critical discussions. Of 59 respondents, only 1 had completed a formal PC rotation.[26] These findings demonstrate that fellows are routinely engaging in PC discussions and assessments without formal instruction or evaluation.

To complement the surveys reported elsewhere in this article, modified questionnaires were sent to the same cohort of fellowship program directors for US gynecologic oncology and hepatopancreaticobiliary/surgical oncology programs.[29,30] PC consult services were available at all included institutions, with inpatient PC available at 96.6% of gynecologic oncology programs and more than 70% of surgical oncology programs. Sixty-three percent of gynecologic oncology program directors and 70% of hepatopancreaticobiliary/surgical oncology program directors responded. Only 15% of hepatopancreaticobiliary/surgical oncology programs gave fellows the opportunity to rotate on the PC consult team; it was not reported what proportion of programs required this rotation. Forty-eight percent of gynecologic oncology program directors reported having a formal PC rotation as a part of their fellowship program, which was reported as mandatory by 28% of programs.[30] However, the finding that only 4 of 103 gynecologic oncology fellows reported completing a PC rotation suggests that fellows are not capitalizing on the option for elective PC rotation and may not be meeting formal PC requirements where mandated.[28,30]

PC education was delivered in several formats; 97% of gynecologic oncology programs had delivered PC training in the form of lectures, with PC content also being explored at journals clubs in 52% of programs, morbidity and mortality conferences in 38%, and other forums such as tumor boards or grand rounds in 55% (**Table 1**).[30] Hepatopancreaticobiliary/surgical oncology programs integrated PC training as formal education less frequently: a mean 14.8% of programs had lectures on PC; 10% to 11% delivered PC education in small groups, self-study, or other forums; and 17.9% of programs formally assessed fellows' PC comprehension with a skills assessment.[29] However, 34.7% of programs acknowledged no formal delivery of PC education (see **Table 1**).

When asked to identify barriers to the implementation of PC education curricula, program directors cited insufficient space for new curricular elements, fellow or faculty discomfort with death and dying, and a cumbersome process required to make curriculum changes as the main reasons for failing to incorporate more EOL education into fellowship program requirements.[29] Although some program directors did not agree that those obstacles were relevant to their program, they are nevertheless important barriers to explore because they highlight the status and prioritization of PC education in surgical oncology fellowship programs. Faculty discomfort with PC and EOL care may reflect the insufficiency of PC exposure and education for practicing surgeons, but it should not hinder trainee education in these fields.

Trainee discomfort with death and dying in the field of oncology, although cited by program directors as a barrier to implementing more formal PC and EOL rotations, represents the ultimate incentive for introducing a formal PC curriculum rather than shying away from it. Furthermore, perceived trainee discomfort was not congruent with the importance trainees placed on learning PC and EOL care skills: 98% of respondents in hepatopancreaticobiliary/surgical oncology programs and 95% of gynecologic oncology fellows reported that learning to provide care for dying patients was important, and 93% of hepatopancreaticobiliary/surgical oncology fellows and 98% of gynecologic oncology respondents believed it was their responsibility to help patients prepare for death.[26,28] If surgical faculty are either uncomfortable or ill-equipped to provide that education, dedicated PC physicians (who were present at all respondent institutions) should be prevailed upon to participate.

In medical oncology fellowships, there has been positive feedback about the impact of a longitudinal monthly seminar series for the duration of the fellowship designed to teach trainees in an interactive setting. The 'Difficult Conversations' seminar series was developed by some of the investigators of the *Oncotalk* and *Oncotalk Teach* programs designed to teach medical oncology trainees about communication in cancer care.[31–33] The instructors noted that the trainees lacked specific communication skills

Table 1
Presence of PC rotations or written curricula and modes of delivery for PC content and skills education and across hepatopancreaticobiliary/surgical oncology and gynecologic oncology fellowship programs in the United States [a]

	Hepatopancreaticobiliary/ Surgical Oncology		Gynecologic Oncology
	Mean[b] (%) ± SD of Programs Reporting Use of Delivery Mode	Range (%)[c]	Programs Reporting Use of Delivery Mode (%)
Modes of education delivery			
Lecture	14.8 ± 4.3	7.1–17.9	97
Small group learning	11.7 ± 4.5	7.1–17.9	
Skills assessment	17.9 ± 4.1	14.3–25.0	
Self-study	10.2 ± 2.5	7.1–14.3	
Journal club			52
Morbidity and mortality conferences			38
Other	11.7 ± 1.7	10.7–14.3	55[d]
None	34.7 ± 4.9	28.5–42.9	
PC rotation available	15		48
Mandatory			28
Elective			20
PC rotation completed	1.7		3.9
Written curriculum	N/R		13.8

[a] *Data from* Larrieux G, Wachi BI, Mirua JT, et al. Palliative Care Training in Surgical Oncology and Hepatobiliary Fellowships: A National Survey of Program Directors. Annals of Surgical Oncology 2015;22:S1181–S86, Lefkowitz C, Sukamvanich P, Claxton R, et al. Needs assessment of palliative care education in gynecologic oncology fellowship: We're not teaching what we think is most important. Gynecologic Oncology 2014;135:255–260.
[b] Program directors reported different modes of education delivery for different items of palliative care education. Mean ± SD was calculated for reported use of education delivery modes across 7 PC skills.
[c] Range represents number of programs reporting use of a given educational delivery mode across 7 PC skills.
[d] Gynecologic oncology programs reported that 'other' modes of education delivery included tumor boards, grand rounds, or interactive teaching sessions.

essential to oncology such as how to give information (including the 'asking before telling' approach), listening without interrupting, and addressing 'feelings before facts.' By scheduling monthly lunchtime workshops, instructors were able to integrate seminars consisting of case discussions, reflective writing, and role-training into the fellows' clinical schedules. Although this stage of the project was intended to assess trainee response to the educational method, the investigators anticipate the project will evolve to include assessing trainee skill acquisition and subsequent behavioral change in real clinical settings.[32]

For oncology trainees, programs like "Difficult Conversations" or *OncoTalk* are especially valuable because the type and extent of discussion fellows have with their patients is very different from medical school or residency. Oncology fellows in both medicine and surgery have to present the risks and benefits of multimodality therapy to their patients, including initiating conversations about lack of treatment effectiveness or anticipated futility of interventions. They must be aware of factors that qualify patients for available clinical trials and be sufficiently informed to discuss trial eligibility. Before fellowship, trainees often do not have access to the resources necessary for expertise in these areas, nor are they aware of institution-specific options for palliative procedures, therapies, clinical trials, and hospice care. A reanimated PC curriculum should therefore be a part of all surgical, medical, and radiation oncology training programs; a firm foundation in the relevant regional, institutional, and oncology-specific considerations is necessary for successful patient care and successful training as a cancer care provider. Furthermore, fellows should be provided with a model of what constitutes excellent care, opportunities for practice, and timely critical evaluation.[33] Given the evidence demonstrating improved patient QOL and quality of care with early PC interventions, as well as the fact that surgical fellows in oncologic disciplines are eager for more EOL education, structuring fellowship programs to include a robust PC curriculum is imperative.

Surgical Practice

Despite the essential role modern surgeons assume in cancer symptom management and EOL care, formal training for practicing surgeons in many facets of PC is lacking. Although more resources and educational opportunities are now available to surgeons looking to pursue advanced PC training, surgeon experts in the field are uncommon. As of 2017, only 69 surgeons were board certified in both surgery and palliative medicine.[34] The literature on improving comprehension of PC principles and helping practicing surgeons incorporate these principles into their clinical care is similarly rare. A 2016 systematic review of educational interventions to train health care professionals in EOL communication identified no studies including attending surgeons or oncologists.[35] A 2002 randomized controlled trial from the UK evaluated the impact of a communication course for oncologists on general communication skills, but did not address PC or EOL care conversations in particular.[36] In a 2018 systematic review of educational models designed to improve either surgeon or anesthetist EOL communication, only 2 publications arising from a single study included attending surgeons.[20] These 2 publications described a novel intervention designed to improve surgeon communication when discussing treatment outcomes with patients over 65 years of age.[37,38] However, surgeon participants were cardiothoracic, vascular, and acute care surgeons; oncology-specific considerations were not explored. These studies focused on a method of communicating surgical outcomes rather than palliative treatment or EOL communication. There is no literature that specifically addresses how we can effectively train busy, practicing surgeons to be facile with PC and EOL care in their oncology practice.

A 2019 quantitative and qualitative analysis evaluated health care providers' understanding of PC principles before and after providers participated in a dedicated PC program taught by palliative medicine physicians.[39] Quantitative analysis was performed based on survey responses. Feedback on how the PC learning intervention impacted health care providers' capacity to provide PC to their patients successfully was elucidated from focus groups and reported as emerging themes. Of the 80 participants, 19 were physicians from the divisions of nephrology, geriatrics, and radiotherapy. Although there were no surgeons in this group, the challenges reported were emblematic of issues encountered by most PC-naïve physicians and surgeons striving to provide quality EOL care. The World Health Organization PC domains examined are displayed in **Table 2**. Providers showed improved understanding of several domains after training, but failed to show improved understanding of PC

Table 2
Assessment of health care provider understanding of fundamental domains of PC before and after focused PC training[a]

WHO PC Domain	Pretraining vs Post-training Score (%)	P value
Domains showing improvement		
Improving patient QOL	23.4 vs 61.0	<.001
Early applicability of PC in illness trajectory	3.9 vs 23.4	<.001
Team approach to addressing needs	7.8 vs 23.4	.006
Helping family to cope during patient illness	10.4 vs 23.4	.016
Psychological aspects of patient care	18.2 vs 44.2	<.001
Spiritual aspects of patient care	2.6 vs 20.8	<.001
Addressing patient and family needs	23.4 vs 53.2	<.001
Treatment of physical symptoms	22.1 vs 40.3	.001
Domains showing no improvement		
Life-threatening illness	53.2 vs 64.9	NS
Prevention and relief of suffering	32.5 vs 28.6	NS
Treatment of pain	33.8 vs 39.0	NS
Helping family cope with bereavement	1.3 vs 7.8	NS
Investigations to improve clinical management	0 vs 0	NS
Encouraging patients to live actively	1.3 vs 9.1	NS
Affirming life	0 vs 2.6	NS

Abbreviations: NS, not significant; WHO, World Health Organization.
[a] *Data from* Artioli A, Bedini G, Bertocchi E, et al. Palliative care training addressed to hospital health care professionals by palliative care specialists: a mixed-method evaluation. BMC Palliative Care 2019;18(88):10.

domains related to life-threatening illness, prevention and relief of suffering, pain management, helping families to cope with bereavement, investigations to improve clinical management, encouraging patients to live actively, and affirming life (**Table 2**). Furthermore, despite improvement, these results show a low level of understanding even after training; the raw percentage of respondents comprehending these principles was poor. Only 2.6% of respondents grew to understand the importance of affirming their patient's life. No respondents had any baseline understanding of, nor developed any understanding of, investigations they could use to identify and improve management of clinical problems in patients at EOL.[39]

As discussed elsewhere in this article, pretest and post-test knowledge after PC educational interventions may not be the most useful outcome. Furthermore, although participants demonstrated improved understanding in some PC domains, post-test scores were still low. This finding may suggest that changes in preintervention and postintervention test results speak more to test-taking ability and retention at the trainee versus practitioner level than true appreciation of the material learned. Additionally, established practitioners may be less open to learning new approaches.

The qualitative analysis was more informative in terms of identifying preconceived barriers to PC provision and discrete changes in participant attitudes after the intervention. Preintervention and postintervention feedback demonstrated that health care providers were able to implement PC strategies more effectively for their patients after participating in training. Specifically, providers reported preintervention that they needed to know how to activate PC provision for their patients outside of hospital, that appropriate timing for PC consultation was unclear, and that there were often discrepancies between PC specialist goals compared with the goals of the attending physician. After training, participants felt better equipped to integrate PC and PC specialists into in-hospital care as well as ensure ongoing care after discharge. They also recognized that their training in EOL communication was lacking and were eager for future education in this domain.[39] With PC now an integral part of care for oncology patients, it is important for cancer care providers to take advantage of the PC specialists in their institution to provide guidance and clarification of resources and avenues for PC provision. Perhaps more important, oncology providers and PC physicians should seek each other out to coordinate educational efforts that will beget a more cohesive EOL care approach for patients.

Regrettably, time constraints may limit the ability of practicing surgeons and other physicians to engage in extensive PC training. To address this, efforts to provide online training resources have increased and their effect was explored in a study of primary care providers who were randomized to an online PC training course intervention or voluntary in-person PC training.[40] There were no significant differences in patient QOL or symptom control between physician groups. However, 86.6% of primary care providers in the intervention group completed the online training, whereas only 13.4% of providers in the control group accessed the in-person course. Given the immense time constraints of a surgical practice, online education may be the most pragmatic method to ensure attending physician access to PC education and encourage training completion. This approach has become even more relevant as efforts to create accessible online education platforms have increased in the context of the COVID-19 pandemic.

Two studies from 2014 and 2016 assessed a statewide PC communication training initiative, the COMFORT course, focusing on 7 modules pertaining to specific aspect of PC communication: Communication, Orientation and options, Mindful communication, Family, Openings, Relating, Team.[41,42] The initial pilot study was administered to physicians, nurses, and other health care providers. It included modules on communication, health literacy, cultural theory, communication with family and caregivers, and team communication including multidisciplinary collaboration and creating collective goals. The 25 physician participants agreed or strongly agreed that the course content was clear and relevant, the instructors knowledgeable, and the teaching effective.[42] This training was then established as a 2-day course covering the 7 communication modules. Fifty-eight delegates from PC programs across California were chosen to both participate in and learn how to administer the curriculum. Nine months after completing the course, the delegates had trained an additional 962 care providers from their home institutions using the COMFORT curriculum, including 151 physicians. Many delegates had incorporated the curriculum into preexisting designated training time, some had made COMFORT training mandatory for new hires on PC or oncology units, and some had incorporated it into orientation materials for residents, fellows, and students completing a PC rotation.[41] These data suggest that online PC resources can be effective for motivated learners at the attending level. It also makes a case for supporting PC or oncology physicians, nurses, or allied health professionals to learn a PC curriculum that can then be brought back to their institutions and integrated into routine oncology training. Although the published COMFORT curriculum was administered in person, it could be adapted for online access or virtual administration. Additional online resources for surgeons in practice seeking foundational learning or additional training in PC are described in the section on resources for palliative care education.

Compass Oncology (previously Northwest Cancer Specialists) of Oregon and southwest Washington developed a seminar series to improve PC awareness and competency.[43] Training administered at pilot sites included seminars on ACP, communication skills, and bereavement. Interdisciplinary clinical care conferences were also implemented. All participants completed ACP directives for themselves to become familiar with the process and foster empathy and comfort with ACP and goals-of-care conversations. After the series, 75% of physicians and nurses reported increased access to patient support and resources.[43] More than one-half of patients had documented ACP conversations in their electronic medical record, and the documentation of advance directives in the electronic medical record increased by 3% over the course of the study. Only 3% of the patients discussed at clinical care conferences received chemotherapy in the last 2 weeks of life.[43] Other access issues were uncovered, such as the location and language of ACP forms in clinic, and insufficient psychosocial resources for patients. These provided targetable areas for improvement such that 2 social workers were hired to enhance support services. These results were mirrored in a state-wide study from Wisconsin designed to improve ACP education by implementing a course for patients and families dedicated to increasing APC conversations and documentation.[44] Although changes were not significant, there were trends toward decreased intensive care unit use and increased ACP documentation on admission, as well as increased recruitment of racial minorities, who are often marginalized and underrepresented in these studies.[44] Although these training interventions were not designated for surgeons specifically, it demonstrates how collaborative institutional efforts can improve literacy, comfort, and familiarity with PC and EOL resources for patients and health care providers, as well as foster a collegial network with cohesive educational goals.

PC resources and guidance available to surgical oncologists vary substantially by region and institution. Surgical oncologists who are unfamiliar with navigating PC systems may be less effective in providing their patients with optimal EOL care, as well as educating and evaluating trainee proficiency in PC and EOL skills. This section has described some options for offering PC training to the practicing surgeon, but creative solutions are still required to make PC literacy ubiquitous across surgical oncologists and ensure that PC education resources are readily available, accessible, and serviceable for surgeons.

RESOURCES FOR PALLIATIVE CARE EDUCATION

Box 1
PC educational resources for trainees

- *Surgical Palliative Care: A Resident's Guide* is intended to make the case for high-quality PC and provide basic knowledge and skills for palliative and EOL care. It was written as part of a PC curriculum project between the American College of Surgeons and Cunniff-Dixon Foundation, named for both the founder's partner and her oncologist. Available at: https://www.facs.org/-/media/files/education/palliativecare/surgicalpalliativecareresidents.ashx. Accessed October 3, 2020.[23]

- Surgeons Educational Self-Assessment Program (SESAP) began including questions pertaining to pain and symptoms management in their 11th edition[45] and have grown to include 20 questions on ethics in the seventeenth edition (most recent). However, only 6 were related to PC and EOL care and communication.[46]

- *OncoTalk* is a teaching model designed for medical oncology trainees to improve communication between care providers and patients with cancer. A chapter describing the method was published in the *Handbook of Communication in Oncology* and PC in 2011.[31]

Box 2
PC educational resources for surgeons in practice

- *Palliative Care* was published in 1997 and serves as an introduction to PC for the practicing surgeon.[47]

- The American College of Surgeons annual Clinical Congress includes panel sessions, town halls, and scientific forum presentations on PC in surgery. The annual Surgical Palliative Care Research Symposium started in 2015.

- *Promoting Excellence in End-of-Life Care* was a national program of the Robert Wood Johnson Foundation and resources for self-study are available for oncology specifically: http://www.promotingexcellence.org/resources/cancer.html.[48]

- Harvard Medical School's Center for Palliative Care offers courses for physicians, nurses, and researchers. The Palliative Care Education and Practice course is designed for PC experts and other specialists who want to improve the PC skills. Course details are provided on their website: https://pallcare.hms.harvard.edu/courses/pcep [49]

- Northwestern University Feinberg School of Medicine created the Education in Palliative & End-of-Life Care Program to teach health care professionals the essential PC clinical competencies as well as ensure that experts have the materials to educate others on PC and EOL care. They have curricula focusing on pediatrics, veterans, and PC in the emergency medicine setting. Access to modules, distance learning materials, and information about their conferences can be found on their website: https://www.bioethics.northwestern.edu/programs/epec/ [50]

- Pallium Canada is a national not-for-profit organization designed to improve the quality of PC and access to PC education. They host 2-day courses for practicing health care professionals for a small fee. These courses focus on all facets of PC from practical approaches to symptom management to handling ACP, requests to hasten death, and spiritual care. Further information on these courses is available via telephone (1-833-888-LEAP) or on their website: https://www.pallium.ca/courses/.[51] In the context of the coronavirus disease 2019 pandemic, Pallium Canada has also created a number of free and publicly available webinars. These discuss PC principles, particular challenges to implementing and ensuring accessibility of PC care in the setting of the current pandemic, and many other valuable topics. Available at: https://www.pallium.ca/pallium-canadas-covid-19-response-resources/.[52]

- The Ian Anderson Continuing Education Program in End-of Life Care was offered by the University of Toronto until 2007. In addition to PC principles and skills, these modules discuss the role of specialists in PC, incorporating quality indicators into palliative practice, applying evidence-based practices into EOL care, and more. Their educational modules are still available online: https://www.cpd.utoronto.ca/endoflife/Modules.htm.[53]

- The End of Life Palliative Education Resource Center is published by the University of Washington and sponsored by the Washington Rural Palliative Care Initiative. It provides online resources including peer-reviewed summaries on fundamental PC topics and "Fast Facts" designed to be used as teaching tools. Resources for PC providers in the setting of the COVID-19 pandemic were recently added to their collection. These are available through the website portal: https://waportal.org/resources/end-life-palliative-education-resource-center.[54]

- *VitalTalk* is a tool intended to improve trainee and practitioner communication in the setting of critical illness and EOL. Online resources include virtual coursework, COVID-19 communication tools, and other options for patients and clinicians. Courses are available to enrollees on the *VitalTalk* website: https://www.vitaltalk.org/. Courses are also available through their mobile app.[55]

Box 3
Accredited PC training programs in North America

- A list of accredited hospice and PC fellowships in the United States for physicians and surgeons who wish to develop a practice in PC is available on the Association of American Medical Colleges Electronic Residency Application Service website: https://services.aamc.org/eras/erasstats/par/display.cfm?NAV_ROW=PAR&SPEC_CD=540.[56]
- A list of accredited programs through the Canadian Society of Palliative Care Physicians including 2-year subspecialty programs and 1-year enhanced skills programs is available at the Canadian Society of Palliative Care Physicians website: http://www.cspcp.ca/information/training-opportunities/.[57]

Box 4
PC evaluation and teaching tools for educators

- The Hospice and Palliative Medicine Competency Workgroup published a toolkit of assessment tools for faculty, fellows, and teams including instruction for application of these assessment tools in different domains of PC. This publication is available online through the American Association of Hospice and Palliative Medicine website: http://aahpm.org/uploads/education/competencies/Toolkit%20Intro%202014.pdf.[58]
- The OncoTalk group created a *Tough Talk* toolbox intended to help identify and overcome common teaching challenges, provide effective feedback to oncology trainees, and motivate participants. This and other resources are available on their website: http://depts.washington.edu/toolbox/toc.html [59]

FUTURE DIRECTIONS

Difficulty implementing significant curricular changes was cited by surgical oncology program directors as a reason not to include formal PC rotations in surgical oncology training. However, PC rotations better prepared fellows for clinical practice, and didactic sessions may be insufficient for practical skill development. A formal PC rotation does not have to consist of a dedicated month on a palliative medicine team; a 1- or 2-week rotation would acquaint fellows with institutional pathways for PC and give them opportunities to participate in inpatient and outpatient PC. A longitudinal rotation consisting of 1 day each month could also be scheduled flexibly around surgical cases and clinics.

Evaluation of PC education programs should use objective outcomes that extend to the patient sphere. Measuring the effectiveness of PC training interventions should go beyond trainee confidence and include outcomes such as patient evaluation of the interaction, congruency between true patient goals and advance directives/goals of care documented in the patient's electronic medical record, effectiveness of multimodal pain control, and quantitative changes in hospice referrals.

Surgical oncologists and palliative medicine physicians should strive to collaborate on training initiatives. These may start as institutional studies, but effective interventions could be translated to regional interdisciplinary education programs for all practitioners and trainees in surgical oncology.

SUMMARY

The value of early and integrated PC in surgical patients with cancer has been demonstrated by many studies showing improved patient-centered outcomes. Educating both surgical oncology trainees and practicing surgeons is necessary to provide optimal EOL care for our unique patient population. Formal clinical experience in PC may be especially valuable for surgical oncology trainees.

Surgeon palliative medicine specialists are uncommon, but all cancer centers with surgical oncology training programs have access to a PC service. Taking advantage of our palliative medicine colleagues' experience and expertise will be invaluable in establishing a generation of surgeons who are facile with the language and skills of PC and EOL care. This collaborative relationship will also engender a generation of surgical oncologists committed to lifelong learning and trainee education in PC. There is an expanding arsenal of PC and EOL care resources both in print and online for trainees and surgeons who are interested in optimizing EOL care for their patients with cancer.

CLINICS CARE POINTS

- Early, integrated PC results in improved patient-centered outcomes.
- Trainee and surgeon confidence in communication skills may not translate into accurate assessment of patient needs and goals.
- Didactic PC education is valuable, but may be insufficient to ensure trainee fluency and expertise in EOL care.
- Practical, clinical outcome measurements are required to evaluate the success of educational interventions.
- Collaborative training efforts between PC specialists, surgeons, oncologists, and allied health professionals improves both educational outcomes and patient outcomes.
- PC and EOL education should be delivered by experts.

DISCLOSURE

The authors have nothing to disclose.

REFERENCES

1. Bakitas M, Lyons KD, Hegel MT, et al. Effects of a palliative care intervention on clinical outcomes in patients with advanced cancer: the project ENABLE II randomized controlled trial. J Am Med Assoc 2009;302(7):741–9.
2. Temel JS, Greer JA, Muzikansky A, et al. Early palliative care for patients with metastatic non–small-cell lung cancer. N Engl J Med 2010;363(8):733–42.
3. Zimmerman C, Swami N, Krzyzanowska M, et al. Early palliative care for patients with advanced cancer: a cluster-randomised controlled trial. Lancet 2014;383: 1721–30.
4. Greer JA, Piri WF, Jackson VA, et al. Effect of early palliative care on chemotherapy use and end-of-life care in patients with metastatic non–small-cell lung cancer. J Clin Oncol 2012;30(4):394–400.
5. Bakitas M, Tosteson TD, Li Zhigang, et al. Early versus delayed initiation of concurrent palliative oncology care: patient outcomes in the ENABLE III randomized controlled trial. J Clin Oncol 2015;33(13):1438–45.
6. Williams MA, Wheeler MS. Palliative care: what is it? Home Healthc Nurse 2001; 19(9):550–7.
7. Sheeham DC, Forman WB. Hospice and palliative care: concepts and practice. Sudbury: Massachusetts Jones and Bartlett Publishers, Inc.; 1996.

8. World Health Organization. WHO Definition of Palliative Care. 2020. Available at: https://www.who.int/ncds/management/palliative-care/introduction/en/.   Accessed September 27, 2020.

9. Weissman DE, Block SD. ACGME requirements for end-of-life training in selected residency and fellowship programs: a status report. Acad Med 2002;77(4): 299–304.

10. National Consensus Conference on Medical Education for Care Near the End of Life. Executive Summary. J Palliat Med 2000;3:88–91.

11. Dickinson GE. Thirty-Five Years of End-of-Life Issues in US Medical Schools. Am J Hosp Palliat Med 2011;28(6):412–7.

12. Horowitz R, Gramling R, Quill T. Palliative Care Education in U.S. Medical schools. Med Educ 2014;48(1):59–66.

13. International Association of Medical Colleges. LCME Accreditation Standards. Available at: http://www.iaomc.org/cs.htm. Accessed September 27, 2020.

14. Turrillas P, Teixeria MJ, Maddocks M. A systematic review of training in symptom management in palliative care within postgraduate medical curriculums. J Pain Symptom Manage 2019;57(1):156–70.

15. Bradley CT, Webb TP, Schmitz CC, et al. Structured teaching versus experiential learning of palliative care for surgical residents. Am J Surg 2010;200:542–7.

16. Klaristenfeld DD, Harrington DT, Miner TJ. Teaching palliative care and end-of-life issues: a core curriculum for surgical residents. Ann Surg Oncol 2007;14(6): 1801–6.

17. Bonnano AM, Kiraly LN, Siegel TR, et al. Surgical palliative care training in general surgery residency: an educational needs assessment. Am J Surg 2019;217: 928–31.

18. Wilson IB, Green ML, Goldman L, et al. Is experience a good teacher? How interns and attending physicians understand patients' choices for end-of-life care. SUPPORT Investigators. Study to Understand Prognoses and Preferences for Outcomes and Risks of Treatments. Med Decis Making 1997;17(2):217–27.

19. Kubi B, Istl AC, Lee KT, et al. Advance care planning in cancer: patient preferences for personnel and timing. JCO Oncol Pract 2020;16(9):e875–83.

20. Bakke KE, Miranda SP, Castillo-Angeles M, et al. Training surgeons and anesthesiologists to facilitate end-of-life conversations with patients and families: a systematic review of existing educational models. J Surg Education 2018;75(3): 702–21.

21. Ballou JH, Brasel KJ. Surgical palliative care education. Surg Clin North Am 2019; 99:1037–49.

22. Dickson RP, Engelberg RA, Back AL, et al. Internal medicine trainee self-assessments of end-of-life communication skills do not predict assessments of patients, families, or clinician-evaluators. J Palliat Med 2012;15(4):418–26.

23. Dunn GP, Martensen R, Weissman D, editors. Surgical palliative care: a resident's guide. Chicago: American College of Surgeons; 2009.

24. Pernar LIM, Peyre SE, Smink DS, et al. Feasibility and Impact of a Case-Based Palliative Care Workshop for General Surgery Residents. J Am Coll Surg 2012; 214:231–6.

25. Raoof M, O'Neill L, Neumayer L, et al. Prospective evaluation of surgical palliative care immersion training for general surgery residents. Am J Surg 2017;214: 378–83.

26. Amini A, Miura JT, Larrieux G, et al. Palliative care training in surgical oncology and hepatobiliary fellowships: a national survey of the fellows. Ann Surg Oncol 2015;22:1761–7.

27. Eskander RN, Osann K, Dickson E, et al. Assessment of palliative care training in gynecologic oncology: a gynecologic oncology fellow research network study. Gynecol Oncol 2014;134(2):379–84.

28. Lesnock JL, Arnold RM, Meyn LA, et al. Palliative care education in gynecologic oncology: a survey of the fellows. Gynecol Oncol 2013;130:431–5.

29. Larrieux G, Wachi BI, Mirua JT, et al. Palliative care training in surgical oncology and hepatobiliary fellowships: a national survey of program directors. Ann Surg Oncol 2015;22:S1181–6.

30. Lefkowitz C, Sukamvanich P, Claxton R, et al. Needs assessment of palliative care education in gynecologic oncology fellowship: we're not teaching what we think is most important. Gynecol Oncol 2014;135:255–60.

31. Arnold RM, Back AT, Baile WF, et al. The Oncotalk model. In: David Kissane BB, Phyllis B, Ilora F, editors. Handbook of communication in oncology and palliative care. Oxford Scholarship Online; 2011. https://doi.org/10.1093/acprof:oso/9780199238361.001.0001.

32. Epner DE, Baile WF. Difficult conversations: teaching medical oncology trainees communication skills one hour at a time. Acad Med 2014;89(4):578–84.

33. Back AL, Arnold RM, Baile WF, et al. Faculty development to change the paradigm of communication skills teaching in oncology. J Clin Oncol 2009;27(7):1137–41.

34. Wancata LM, Hinshaw DB, Suwanabol PA. Palliative care and surgical training: are we being trained to be unprepared? Ann Surg 2017;265(1):32–3.

35. Chung H-O, Oczkowski SJW, Hanvey L, et al. Educational interventions to train healthcare professionals in end-of-life communication: a systematic review and meta-analysis. BMC Med Educ 2016;16:131.

36. Fallowfield L, Jenkins V, Farewell V, et al. Efficacy of a Cancer Research UK communication skills training model for oncologists: a randomised controlled trial. Lancet 2002;359:650–6.

37. Kruser JM, Taylor IJ, Campbell TC, et al. "Best Case/Worst Case": training surgeons to use a novel communication tool for high-risk acute surgical problems. J Pain Symptom Manage 2017;53(4):711–9.

38. Taylor IJ, Nabozny MJ, Steffens NM, et al. A framework to improve surgeon communication in high-stakes surgical decisions: best case/worst case. JAMA Surg 2017;152(6):531–8.

39. Artioli A, Bedini G, Bertocchi E, et al. Palliative care training addressed to hospital healthcare professionals by palliative care specialists: a mixed-method evaluation. BMC Palliat Care 2019;18(88):10.

40. Pelayo-Alvarez M, Perez-Hoyos S, Agra-Varela Y. Clinical effectiveness of online training in palliative care of primary care physicians. J Palliat Med 2013;16(10):1188–96.

41. Wittenberg E, Ferrell B, Goldsmith J, et al. Assessment of a statewide palliative care team training course: COMFORT Communication for Palliative Care Teams. J Palliat Med 2016;19(7):746–52.

42. Wittenberg-Lyles E, Goldsmith J, Ferrell B, et al. Assessment of an Interprofessional Online Curriculum for Palliative Care Communication Training. J Palliat Med 2014;17(4):400–6.

43. Hedlund S. Northwest Cancer Specialists (NCS) cares: coordinated, advocacy, resources, education, and support: a palliative care program in an outpatient oncology practice. Omega (Westport) 2013;67(1–2):109–13.

44. Peltier WL, Gani F, Blissitt J, et al. Initial experience with "honoring choices Wisconsin": implementation of an advance care planning pilot in a tertiary care setting. J Palliat Med 2017;20(9):998–1003.
45. Palliative Care Working Group. Office of promoting excellence in end-of-life care: Surgeons' Palliative Care Workgroup report from the field. J Am Coll Surg 2003; 197(4):661–87.
46. American College of Surgeons - Division of Education. Surgical Education and Self-Assessment Program 17. USA, 2019.
47. Milch RA, Dunn GP. The surgeon and palliative care. Bull Am Coll Surg 1997; 82:15–8.
48. Robert Wood Johnson Foundation. Promoting Excellence in End-of-Life Care. 2009. Available at: http://www.promotingexcellence.org/resources/cancer.html. Accessed October 3, 2020.
49. Center for Palliative Care, Harvard Medical School. Palliative Care Education and Practice (PCEP). The President and Fellows of Harvard College 2020. Available at: https://pallcare.hms.harvard.edu/courses/pcep. Accessed October 13, 2020.
50. Northwestern University Feinberg School of Medicine. EPEC: education in palliative and end-of-life care 2020. Available at: https://www.bioethics.northwestern.edu/programs/epec/. Accessed October 13, 2020.
51. Pallium Canada. Our courses 2020. Available at: https://www.pallium.ca/courses/. Accessed October 7, 2020.
52. Pallium Canada. COVID-response: palliative care resources 2020. Available at: https://www.pallium.ca/pallium-canadas-covid-19-response-resources/. Accessed October 7, 2020.
53. Ian Anderson Program, University of Toronto. Ian Anderson Continuing Education Program in End-of Life Care. 2007. Available at: https://www.cpd.utoronto.ca/endoflife/Modules.htm. Accessed October 7, 2020.
54. University of Washington. End of life palliative education resource center 2018. Available at: https://waportal.org/resources/end-life-palliative-education-resource-center. Accessed October 7, 2020.
55. VitalTalk. VitalTalk 2020. Available at: https://www.vitaltalk.org/. Accessed October 10, 2020.
56. Association of American Medical Colleges. Electronic Residency Application Service. 2020. Available at: https://services.aamc.org/eras/erasstats/par/display.cfm?NAV_ROW=PAR&SPEC_CD=540. Accessed October 3, 2020.
57. Canadian Society of Palliative Care Physicians. Training opportunities. 2020. Available at: http://www.cspcp.ca/information/training-opportunities/. Accessed October 7, 2020.
58. HPM Competencies Project Workgroup. Hospice and palliative medicine competencies project: toolkit of assessment methods. Glenview (IL): American Academy of Hospice and Palliative Medicine; 2010.
59. Fryer-Edwards K, Back AR, Baile WF, et al. Tough talk: helping doctors approach difficult conversations. Oncotalk Project. Available at: http://depts.washington.edu/toolbox/toc.html. Accessed October 10, 2020.

Moving?

Make sure your subscription moves with you!

To notify us of your new address, find your **Clinics Account Number** (located on your mailing label above your name), and contact customer service at:

Email: journalscustomerservice-usa@elsevier.com

800-654-2452 (subscribers in the U.S. & Canada)
314-447-8871 (subscribers outside of the U.S. & Canada)

Fax number: 314-447-8029

Elsevier Health Sciences Division
Subscription Customer Service
3251 Riverport Lane
Maryland Heights, MO 63043

*To ensure uninterrupted delivery of your subscription, please notify us at least 4 weeks in advance of move.